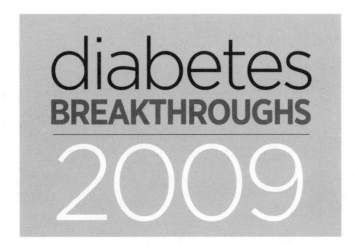

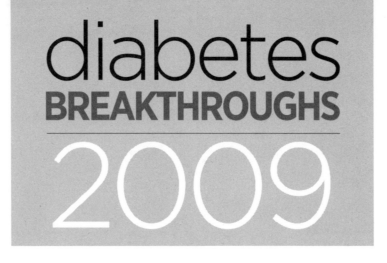

diabetes BREAKTHROUGHS 2009

EXPERT ANSWERS & ADVICE

FROM THE EDITORS OF **Prevention**®

RODALE

© 2009 by Rodale Inc.

All rights reserved. No part of this publication may be reproduced or transmitted in any form or by any means,
electronic or mechanical, including photocopying, recording, or any other information storage and retrieval system,
without the written permission of the publisher.

Prevention is a registered trademark of Rodale Inc.

Printed in the United States of America
Rodale Inc. makes every effort to use acid-free ♾, recycled paper ♲.

Photograph credits are on page 349.

Book design by Joanna Williams

Pages 9 to 15 in Chapter 1 were reprinted with permission from the National Women's Health Resource Center.
Copyright 2008 National Women's Health Resource Center, Inc. (NWHRC). All rights reserved.
Visit the NWHRC online at www.healthywomen.org or call toll-free 877-986-9472.

ISBN-13 978–1–60529–974–7
ISBN-10 1–60529–974–X

2 4 6 8 10 9 7 5 3 1 hardcover

We inspire and enable people to improve their lives and the world around them
For more of our products visit **rodalestore.com** or call 800-848-4735

contents

part 3
lose weight

part 4
move it

part 5
stress less

part 6
avoid complications

part 7
diabetes cookbook

THE FUTURE
LOOKS BRIGHT

t's an exciting time to be reporting on diabetes care. Like a locomotive charging downhill, faster, *faster*, **faster**, the medical breakthroughs to ease—and improve—the lives of people with diabetes are coming with astonishing speed. Less-painful testing, more-effective treatments, less-restrictive diets, more hope for a cure—it all adds up to a bright future for people with diabetes.

We've packed this book full of all the latest news and information on diabetes prevention and treatment to help you live your best life in spite of diabetes. In Part 1, Take Control, you'll find a primer to help you better understand diabetes and better explain it to your family and friends. You'll learn about diabetes testing and how to make the most of this important part of your life with this condition. And you'll discover 10 ways to save thousands of dollars on your health care.

We've come a long way since Scottish physician John Rollo put his patients on the first diabetes diet, an "animal diet" of "plain blood puddings" back in 1797! Today, there's no set "diabetes diet" at all, just the best eating plan for you. Part 2, Eat Right, will help you to create it. You'll be eager to make over your grocery cart after reading about the healthiest carb you're not eating, eight foods to eat every day, and the 10 best foods you've been missing out on.

In Part 3, Lose Weight, you'll find tips to help pare down the pounds if you need to. You'll create a weight loss plan that's yours and yours alone. You'll learn how to navigate two of the biggest weight loss minefields: weekends and vacations. And you'll uncover 10 surprising reasons why you may not be losing weight even if you're doing everything right.

Way back in 1916, doctors established the connection between exercise and diabetes treatment. In Part 4, Move It, you'll find the best ways to get moving, with our walking workout for people with diabetes and our ultimate exercise plan to keep your heart healthy, your bones strong, your mind sharp, and your skin glowing. Plus, try three gentle, but effective, ways to work out—dance, yoga, and tai chi.

Life is stressful, and living with a chronic condition even more so. That's why we've dedicated Part 5 to help you Stress Less. Here you'll find the best Zen for you, read about the importance of resilience, and discover nine foods that can help your mood.

In Part 6, you'll learn how to Avoid Complications. Diabetes is a risk factor for heart disease and cancer, which is why these two conditions are discussed here in great detail. You'll also learn why uncontrolled blood sugar can cause wrinkles, and five steps to help ensure that it won't.

Part 7, the Diabetes Cookbook, offers more than 100 nutritious, but more important, delicious, meals and snacks to help fight diabetes—for example, Almond-Pecan Waffles, Candy-like Almonds, Mocha Custard, and many more, both good and good for you. Bon appétit!

We hope all these medical breakthroughs, prevention tips, and treatment techniques will help you make your '09 simply divine.

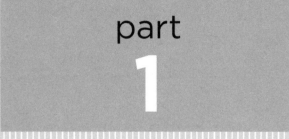

part

1

TAKE
CONTROL

medical BREAKTHROUGHS

Here's the latest and greatest diabetes research to help you take control.

MAKE A CHANGE

Receiving a diagnosis such as diabetes can be crushing. But results from a new study are empowering. Researchers at the University of Leicester in the United Kingdom reviewed more than 20 studies that had previously been conducted on 8,084 people with prediabetes. The researchers found that lifestyle changes, such as exercising and losing weight, were at least as effective as drug therapy in delaying or preventing type 2 diabetes. Interestingly, the review suggested that lifestyle changes had the greatest impact on the people who were the most overweight.

"Based on these findings, people with prediabetes should seek further advice on how they can improve their health, as simple lifestyle changes in terms of diet and exercise have been shown to significantly reduce the risk of progressing to type 2 diabetes," says study author Clare Gillies, PhD.

BUTT OUT

No doubt, this isn't the first time you've read this: If you smoke, quit. But we felt compelled to say it again in light of a recent study. Researchers in Switzerland found that smoking increases insulin resistance and is associated with gaining fat in your midsection. As a result, smoking increases the risk for metabolic syndrome and diabetes.

If you're on the other end of the lit cig, you're not faring much better. In another study, researchers in Japan found that people who were exposed to passive smoke at work had an increased risk of diabetes. So snuff out those cigarettes!

MAKE YOUR PILLBOX WORK FOR YOU

Forget to take your meds again? Now, an interactive pillbox can gently remind you—and even by cell phone, fax, or pager—if anything's amiss. The new Med-eMonitor (an electronic box that hooks up to a standard phone jack) announces medication time with a musical tone, along with warnings about potential food or drug interactions. If you fail to confirm that you've taken your dose, you're notified after 3 minutes. Research has shown that patients who use the device take their meds more than 90 percent of the time (about $60 per month; www.informedix.com).

SEARCH FOR A CURE

Scientists have successfully implanted monkeys with insulin-creating cells derived from the pancreas of a pig. Researchers at the Washington University School of Medicine in St. Louis predict they'll soon have the ability to cure diabetes in monkeys using this procedure; they hope to begin conducting human trials in the next few years.

Farther out on the horizon, some researchers are considering gastrointestinal bypass surgery as a possible treatment for diabetes. Researchers at Weill Cornell Medical College of Cornell University–New York Presbyterian Hospital in New York City conducted a review of studies of obese people with diabetes who had undergone gastrointestinal bypass procedures and found it to be effective in actually curing type 2 diabetes.

Although the researchers aren't sure why it is helpful, the prevailing theory is that the surgery creates changes in hormone signaling from the small bowel.

BREATHE EASY

Chemists at the University of California, Irvine, are developing a breath test to monitor sugar levels in people with diabetes. The pinprick-free technique measures the level of methyl nitrates in exhaled air, which is much higher in hyperglycemic individuals.

WATCH OUT FOR RX WARNINGS

Since the Food and Drug Administration (FDA) slapped a "black box" label on the diabetes drug Avandia in May 2007, three other remedies have received the warning, which indicates the potential for life-threatening side effects. Here's what *Prevention* advisor and public health expert David Katz, MD, says you should do if one of your medications gets flagged.

Q: A drug I've taken for years was just given a black box warning. Should I stop taking it?

A: Not without talking to your doctor first. Consider the risks of not taking a prescription: Avandia, for example, may slightly raise your chances of heart disease, but if your diabetes goes out of control without it, guess what? That dramatically increases your danger. Plus, your doctor should already be aware of the drug's risks. By the time there's enough evidence to warrant a black box, the research behind it should not come as a surprise. Ask your doctor if he thinks the benefits outweigh the risks for you. If he can't tell you why he's prescribing a specific drug, you have every right to not be comfortable taking it.

Q: How will my doctor really know what's best for me?

A: Your doctor will base his decision partly on your medical records and family history, but you also need to tell him what other drugs you're taking (both prescription and over the counter), plus any vitamins or supplements.

Q: Could I be using a black box drug without knowing it?

A: Yes. You won't typically see the warning on a bottle of pills. The black box—actually just a thick black border around text—appears within the accompanying printed materials.

Your doctor may not pay close attention, either. In one study, physicians prescribed drugs without following black-boxed instructions about half the time, mostly neglecting tests that should be performed first.

Q: These warnings are serious! Why are the drugs still used?

A: Because the remedies are a good option for many patients. Realize that if America regulated automobiles the way it regulates medications, cars would all come with these warnings; their potential for injury is very high. Black boxes alert doctors to circumstances in which a drug may be inappropriate—even though for others, its benefits trump the risks.

DON'T GO TOO LOW

Some medications can cause dangerously low blood sugar. If you are taking any of the drugs on the following list, ask your doctor what you should do to monitor your glucose levels. Also find out what to do if your numbers drop too low.

Glimepiride (Amaryl)

Glipizide (Glucotrol)

Glyburide (Micronase, Glynase, DiaBeta, or the combination drug Glucovance)

Insulin (any injected, pump, or inhaled form)

Nateglinide (Starlix)

Repaglinide (Prandin)

SCRUB UP BEFORE SUGAR TESTS

When it's time to test your blood glucose, be sure you lather up before you prick your finger. The Centers for Disease Control and Prevention recommends washing hands before and after dealing with a cut, which is essentially what you're creating when you perform a blood sugar test.

Use warm water to increase the circulation to your hands, making it easier to get a good sample on the first try. Hand washing can also remove any dirt or food residue that could skew your test results.

SCHEDULE ANOTHER A1C TEST

No doubt, you're swamped like everyone else. But make the time for an A1c test (short for "glycated hemoglobin A1c") every 3 to 6 months. If you're due for one, call and schedule it right away. The A1c test yields an average of what your blood glucose level has been for the past 3 months and shows how your current treatment program is working. The A1c target for most people with diabetes is less than 7 percent. Because the normal range is between 4.2 and 4.3 percent, however, some doctors recommend that people with diabetes aim for 6.5 percent.

If yours is higher, your doctor will work with you to modify your current diabetes care plan so you can get your number down.

GIVE YOURSELF SOME TLC

When people with diabetes have colds or other illnesses totally unrelated to their diabetes, their blood sugar levels commonly rise. That's the case even if they're not eating as much as usual. Being sick is stressful to the body, and any kind of stress can cause sugar levels to rise.

What can you do? First, follow your doctor's advice to treat your cold or illness. But be sure to take care of your diabetes, too. Here's how.

- Continue to monitor your glucose levels. You may even want to test more often than normal if your numbers are running high.
- Keep taking your diabetes medications, even if you're not eating very much.
- Call your doctor if your blood glucose levels are 300 milligrams per deciliter (mg/dL) or higher.

FIND A NEW DIABETES DOCTOR?

It turns out that there may be a greater difference between male doctors and female doctors for diabetes than the letter "s" that differentiates "he" and "she." Researchers in Germany studied more than 50,000 people with diabetes. They found that female doctors provided an overall better quality of care and especially excelled at managing their patients' risk factors. In particular, the patients of female doctors had better glucose control and took fewer oral antidiabetic drugs than did the patients of male doctors.

"Based on these findings, if a person with diabetes is considering changing doctors, he or she might want to choose a female doctor," says study researcher Ioanna Gouni-Berthold, MD.

JOIN THE CLUB

Humans are social creatures by nature. A funny movie, a good cry, and a bottle of wine are all often better when shared with a friend. Add to that list diabetes support. Researchers in Belgium wondered whether or not belonging to a patient support group leads to better diabetes control. They recruited 323 people with type 1 diabetes and 494 people with type 2 diabetes. Although the people had similar blood pressure, cholesterol levels, body mass index, and socioeducational status, the researchers found that the people who belonged to diabetes support groups had better control of their blood glucose.

chapter 1

YOUR LIVING-WITH-DIABETES PRIMER

Use this handy guide to better understand
your diabetes . . . and better explain it
to your family and friends

Much of the food we eat is broken down by digestive juices into a simple sugar called glucose, which is the body's main source of energy. Glucose passes into the bloodstream and, from there, into cells, which use it for energy.

However, most cells require the hormone insulin to "unlock" them so glucose can enter. Insulin is normally produced by beta cells in the pancreas, which is a large gland located behind the stomach. In healthy people, the process of eating signals the pancreas to produce the right amount of insulin to enable the glucose from the food to get into cells. If this process fails or doesn't work properly, however, diabetes develops.

In people with diabetes, the pancreas produces little or no insulin, or the body's cells do not respond to the insulin that is produced. As a result, glucose builds up in the blood, overflows into the urine, and passes out of the body. Thus, the body loses its main source of fuel even though the blood contains large amounts of glucose.

TYPES OF DIABETES

There are several types of diabetes: type 1, type 2, and gestational. We'll talk about each in turn.

Type 1 (Insulin-Dependent) Diabetes

In type 1 diabetes, the pancreas makes little or no insulin because the insulin-producing beta cells have been destroyed. Type 1 diabetes is less common than type 2 diabetes, accounting for about 5 to 10 percent of diabetes cases. Although this disorder was formerly known as "juvenile diabetes," and typically develops during childhood or young adulthood, it can appear at any age.

Type 1 diabetes is classified as an autoimmune disease, which is a condition that results when the immune system turns against a specific part or system of the body. With type 1 diabetes, the immune system attacks and destroys the insulin-producing beta cells in the pancreas. Scientists do not know exactly what causes the body's immune system to attack the beta cells, but they believe that both genetic and environmental factors are involved.

Type 2 (Non-Insulin-Dependent) Diabetes

In type 2 diabetes, the pancreas makes insulin, but the body does not respond to it properly. (This is called insulin resistance.) In time, the pancreas can fail to produce enough of its own insulin, and it will require insulin replacement. Type 2 diabetes most often occurs in adults older than age 30, but it may also develop in younger people. Factors that contribute to insulin resistance and type 2 diabetes are genetics, obesity, physical inactivity, and advancing age.

Type 2 diabetes is on the rise in the United States, and rates are expected to continue to go up, according to the Centers for Disease Control and Prevention. One reason is the increasing prevalence of obesity among Americans. Another reason is the relatively low levels of physical activity among American adults. (More than half of us, 60 percent, don't get enough physical activity.) Other factors include the increasing age of the population and the fast growth rate of certain ethnic populations that are at high risk for developing the condition, including Latino and Hispanic Americans.

Q&A

Will I need to take insulin to treat my type 2 diabetes?

For type 2 diabetes, as long as your body is making enough insulin, you won't need insulin injections. Sometimes, lifestyle modifications are sufficient to keep type 2 under control in the early years, but many types of medications can help people with type 2 diabetes lower their blood sugar by stimulating insulin production, decreasing the amount of sugar made by the liver, slowing starch absorption, and boosting insulin sensitivity. Your health care professional may recommend a combination of two of these drugs or one of these drugs plus insulin.

Is there any way to take insulin that doesn't involve needles?

Yes, but it is expensive. The FDA has approved insulin jet injectors, which look like large pens and send a fine spray of insulin through the skin by a high-pressure air mechanism. Insulin jet injectors are costly, so try out several models before you purchase one. Also ask your doctor about other insulin-delivery options, such as insulin pens and pumps. Newer methods are currently in development, such as nasal sprays.

Gestational (Pregnancy) Diabetes

A third type of diabetes, gestational diabetes, is one of the most common problems of pregnancy. Left uncontrolled, it can be dangerous for both the mother and the baby. Gestational diabetes results when hormones produced by the placenta increase the mother's resistance to insulin. This resistance usually disappears when the pregnancy ends, but women who have had gestational diabetes have a greater risk of developing type 2 diabetes later in life. Pregnant women are routinely screened for gestational diabetes between their 24th and 28th weeks.

Prediabetes

A new term, *prediabetes*, describes an increasingly common condition in which blood glucose levels are higher than normal but not high enough for a diagnosis of diabetes. About 41 million Americans between the ages of 40 and 74 have prediabetes.

People with prediabetes have impaired fasting glucose (100 to 125 milligrams per deci-liter [mg/dL] after an overnight fast), or they have impaired glucose tolerance as indicated by one or more simple tests used to measure glucose levels. The American Diabetes Association (ADA) reports that in one study, about 11 percent of people with prediabetes developed type 2 diabetes each year during the average 3 years of follow-up. Other research shows that most people with this condition go on to develop type 2 diabetes within 10 years unless they make modest changes in their diet and level of physical activity.

Some long-term damaging effects to the body, particularly to the heart and circulatory system, may start during the prediabetes phase of the disease.

MANAGING DIABETES

You can effectively control and manage diabetes once it has been accurately diagnosed. The goal of diabetes management, according to the American Association of Clinical Endocrinologists, is to prevent short- and long-term complications of diabetes from developing.

Without proper management, people with diabetes can develop serious or deadly complications from high glucose levels, including blindness, kidney disease, and nerve damage, as well as vascular disease that can lead to amputations, heart disease, and strokes. Uncontrolled diabetes can complicate pregnancy; birth defects are also more common in babies born to women with uncontrolled diabetes.

For people with type 1 diabetes, controlling blood sugar levels usually means getting three to four (and sometimes more) shots of insulin a day, adjusting doses to food and exercise, testing blood glucose up to eight times a day depending on their health care provider's recommendations, and adhering to a planned diet.

Type 2 diabetes may be controlled initially by a planned diet, exercise, and daily monitoring of glucose levels. Frequently, oral drugs that lower blood glucose levels or insulin injections need to be added to this regimen.

Treating diabetes comprehensively—that is, managing not only blood glucose but also blood pressure and cholesterol—is crucial to helping prevent heart attacks and stroke.

The good news is that people with diabetes who maintain lower blood glucose, blood pressure, and cholesterol levels can lower their risk of cardiovascular disease. To reduce your risk, follow the "ABC" approach recommended by the National Diabetes Education Program, the National Institutes of Health (NIH), and the ADA. The ABCs are easy to remember:

A stands for the A1c test (short for "glycated hemoglobin A1c"), which measures average blood glucose over the previous 2 to 3 months

B is for blood pressure

C is for cholesterol

Diabetes treatment guidelines issued by the American College of Physicians (ACP) emphasize the importance of aggressive blood pressure control in lowering the risk for heart disease, stroke, and early death in people with type 2 diabetes. Prior to these guidelines, most of the focus in diabetes care had been on tightly controlling blood sugar, but new evidence suggests that both blood sugar and blood pressure are very important in managing the disease.

The ADA and the NIH recommend that people with diabetes and high blood pressure strive for blood pressure levels of less than 130/80 millimeters of mercury (mm Hg). The ACP recommends both thiazide diuretics and angiotensin-converting enzyme (ACE) inhibitors as first-line agents to control blood pressure in most people with diabetes.

> The times more likely that a man will develop diabetes if he has low testosterone, regardless of body mass, according to the Third National Health and Nutrition Examination Survey: 4 times

SEEKING TREATMENT

Developing a chronic disease is not your fault, although many people who develop type 2 diabetes may feel this way, especially when obesity is an issue. If you are diagnosed with diabetes, it is essential that you receive comprehensive information—whether from a primary health care professional, a certified diabetes educator, or an endocrinologist—on

Women and Diabetes: Special Concerns

In the United States, 9.7 million women age 20 and older have diabetes. Here are some particular health issues of concern for women with diabetes.

Heart disease: Women with diabetes develop heart disease more often than other women, and their heart disease is more severe. Women younger than age 50 with diabetes are more vulnerable to heart attacks and strokes than those without diabetes, because the disease seems to cancel the protective effects of estrogen on a woman's heart prior to menopause. Women with diabetes are also at even greater risk for developing heart disease after menopause.

According to the National Cholesterol Education Program from the National Heart, Lung, and Blood Institute (NHLBI), diabetes poses as great a risk for a person having a heart attack in 10 years as heart disease itself and should be managed just as aggressively. Heart disease and stroke are the major causes of death for people with diabetes. In fact, approximately two-thirds of people with diabetes die from cardiovascular disease.

Cholesterol levels: Women with diabetes have lower levels of high-density lipoprotein (HDL) cholesterol (the "good" cholesterol) and higher levels of triglycerides, or fats, in the blood. According to the NHLBI's cholesterol management guidelines, elevated low-density lipoprotein (LDL) cholesterol (the "bad" cholesterol that contributes to plaque buildup in your arteries) is a major cause of coronary heart disease and should be treated aggressively. Although LDL levels are not higher in women with diabetes, studies find that reducing LDL levels to less than 100 mg/dL can help prevent heart attacks and strokes in women with diabetes. High cholesterol is typically treated with specially designed diets low in saturated fat, weight loss programs, exercise, and, if necessary, medication.

High blood pressure: The ideal blood pressure for people with diabetes is less than 130/80 mm Hg, according to the American Diabetes Association.

Urinary tract and vaginal infections: Urinary tract infections (UTIs) and yeast infections are more common in women with diabetes. The fungi and bacteria that cause these infections thrive in a high-sugar environment, and the body's immune system can't fight them as effectively when blood glucose levels are too high.

how to manage your condition and avoid complications. People with diabetes also need to regularly review and revise their strategies for managing their disease, under the guidance of health care professionals.

The percentage of people with diabetes who do not know whether they have type 1 or type 2: 17 percent

People with diabetes should be seen regularly by health care professionals who monitor their diabetes and check for complications. Health care professionals who specialize in diabetes are called endocrinologists or diabetologists. In addition, people with diabetes often see ophthalmologists for eye examinations, podiatrists for routine foot care, dietitians for help in planning meals, and diabetes educators for instruction in day-to-day care.

Living with diabetes can be overwhelming at times. Like all chronic diseases, it affects every aspect of your daily routine. Diabetes management is not as simple as just taking a pill. It requires timing of meals, checking blood sugar, and being vigilant about exercise, all in accordance with a personalized management plan developed in consultation with health care professionals.

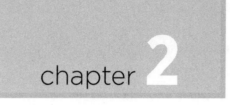

chapter 2

TESTING 1-2-3

Use this guidebook to help you get the most out of
tests, track your progress, and stay healthy

Testing is a very important part of your diabetes care program. In this chapter, you'll learn how to make the most of the information you get from glucose testing. You'll also find some handy worksheets to record your results. But that's not the only test you need for improving your overall well-being. Read on for information about additional ways to monitor your health from head to toe, including cholesterol tests, blood pressure screenings, and examinations of the eyes and feet.

GLUCOSE TESTING

Blood glucose values are a bit like the stock market: Although they generally follow a trend, they can bounce around from day to day. Certain situations can trigger an unexpected rise. Any sort of illness or infection can boost your blood glucose; even a minor upper respiratory illness or a scraped foot can cause a significant jump in your numbers. Stress can too, due to the action of stress-related hormones.

Having some up-and-down swings in blood sugar is normal, but if your glucose remains high day after day, it will increase your risk of medical complications. By the same token, too-low sugar can also be extremely dangerous. Talk with your doctor about either situation—whether your blood sugar is too high or too low. You should also talk with your doctor before you make any changes to your diet and exercise habits. That's because as you begin a healthful diet and exercise program, your numbers are likely to fall significantly.

Use the following guidelines to make sure you're testing often enough.

If you have type 1 diabetes or are using insulin for type 2 or gestational diabetes, check your glucose at least three times a day or according to the schedule your doctor recommends.

If you have type 2 diabetes and are using oral medications, there is no optimal testing frequency. As a rule of thumb, however, when your diet, medications, exercise routine, or health status changes, test more frequently.

Regular glucose testing is especially important if you are taking diabetes medications, particularly insulin or medications that cause your body to release insulin. These powerful drugs actively push your blood sugar down. The combination of drugs, diet, and exercise may end up pushing it too low.

As you're testing, it's important to keep track of your blood sugar. An easy way to do this is to use a logbook or a simple chart like the one on page 22.

HEMOGLOBIN A1C TESTING

Your blood glucose test will tell you how you're doing at the moment you take the test, but how about tracking your health over the long haul? The main method for assessing your progress and treatment over a period of several months is the A1c test (short for "glycated hemoglobin A1c"). The higher your A1c levels, the greater your risk of circulatory problems. Evidence suggests that keeping A1c low is particularly important for the health of your eyes and kidneys.

Your A1c level should be checked every 6 months, or every 3 months if your diet, medications, or general health is changing or if previous values have been too high. If your A1c is high, your doctor will be concerned, and you should be, too. If it is low, you are doing well. The American Diabetes Association (ADA) says that A1c should be less than 7 percent, and for people for whom further reductions are possible, it should be closer to 6 percent. Unfortunately, only a small number of people with diabetes in the United States manage to achieve A1c levels under 7 percent.

A typical oral diabetes medication brings down A1c by an average of 1 point, or a bit less. The effect of a good diet on A1c varies depending on how good your control is when you start, how well you follow the diet, and how much excess weight you lose. Your result will also be affected by exercise, genetics, and other factors.

CHOLESTEROL TESTING

Your doctor should check your cholesterol at regular intervals, at least once a year. High levels of cholesterol in the blood can damage your heart, major blood pathways, and the delicate blood vessels of the eyes and kidneys. Here are the numbers to aim for.

Total cholesterol: According to the US government's National Cholesterol Education Program, total cholesterol should be below 200 milligrams per deciliter (mg/dL) (5.2 millimoles per liter [mmol/L]). You should aim for a considerably lower goal, however. Large population studies have shown that the lower your cholesterol, the lower your risk of heart problems, until you reach a threshold of about 150 mg/dL (3.9 mmol/L). Use that as your target, not the more permissive "official" figure.

Low-density lipoprotein cholesterol (LDL): LDL cholesterol is often called "bad" cholesterol because it raises your risk of heart problems and other blood vessel complications. According to the US government, your LDL should be below 100 mg/dL (2.6 mmol/L) if you have diabetes. But many scientists are pushing for stricter standards, including reductions to below 70 mg/dL (1.8 mmol/L) for high-risk patients. Some authorities recommend lowering your LDL by 30 to 40 percent regardless of what your starting level is. Your risk of heart problems drops as LDL decreases, until you reach a level of approximately 40 mg/dL (1.0 mmol/L).

High-density lipoprotein cholesterol (HDL): HDL cholesterol is often called "good" cholesterol because it carries cholesterol out of the body. Generally speaking, the higher your HDL, the better. Current recommendations are to have an HDL level above 45 mg/dL (1.2 mmol/L) for men and above 55 mg/dL (1.4 mmol/L) for women.

Some doctors, however, interpret HDL in the context of your total cholesterol concentration: In that case, a favorable HDL reading would be at least one-third of your total cholesterol. For example, if your total cholesterol is 150, a healthy HDL would be 50 or above. This is an important consideration, because many people who follow healthful diets do not have much of any kind of cholesterol.

Triglycerides: Triglycerides are tiny fat particles transported in the bloodstream. Normal triglyceride concentration is less than 150 mg/dL (3.9 mmol/L). Keeping below this number can help prevent heart disease.

OTHER TESTS YOU SHOULDN'T MISS

Ask your doctor to run other tests to track your progress. The following are three common but important ones.

Complete blood count (CBC): This test shows the state of your blood cells. Many people with diabetes develop anemia, meaning they have fewer red blood cells than they should. A CBC lets your doctor easily check this. If your blood count is low, your doctor will investigate the reasons for it, which could include kidney disease, iron deficiency, use of certain medications, abnormal bleeding, or other factors.

Chemistry panel: A routine chemistry panel assesses your overall health, with a special focus on your kidneys and liver. This test lets doctors check for potential adverse effects caused by medications.

Don't despair if any of your laboratory values are not where they should be. Consider it a reason to take action. You will want to optimize your diet and work with your doctor to plot a course for tracking the effectiveness of your overall health regimen.

Blood pressure: Maintaining healthy blood pressure is extremely important. As you can imagine, increased pressure inside your arteries can damage the arteries themselves, as well as your heart, eyes, kidneys, and nerves. The longer your blood pressure stays high, the more damage it can do.

Problems can travel in the other direction, too. Damage to the kidneys can *lead* to high blood pressure. The reason is that your kidneys play an important role in regulating your blood pressure, and if they have been assaulted by diabetes, they can lose some of their ability to do this. Here are your targets.

Normal blood pressure is less than 120/80 millimeters of mercury (mm Hg). Most doctors want to keep the blood pressure of people with diabetes under 130/80 mm Hg. If you have kidney-related problems or any other complication, the goal will be stricter, typically 125/75 mm Hg.

Have your blood pressure checked regularly. If it is not where it should be, take another look at your diet and speak with your doctor about what, if any, additional treatments you may need.

CHECKING YOUR TOTAL-BODY HEALTH

Because diabetes affects your whole body, it's important to keep an eye out for specific concerns and complications. Here are a few body parts you need to pay special attention to.

Kidneys: Because your kidneys can easily be affected by diabetes, your doctor will check your kidney health with a simple urine test at least once a year. The goal is to see whether your kidneys are losing protein—specifically a protein molecule called albumin. Albumin itself is not especially important. But if it shows up in your urine, it is a sign that your kidneys have been affected by diabetes and are not holding on to albumin as they should. Albumin losses of greater than 30 milligrams over 24 hours are considered abnormal.

Your doctor will also check your blood for creatinine and estimate your glomerular filtration rate. Don't worry; he or she will interpret the results of these tests for you.

Eyes: At least once a year, you should schedule an eye examination with an ophthalmologist to check for any sign of retinopathy. These changes cannot be detected by an ordinary eye examination with a doctor's ophthalmoscope or during an optometric examination for eyeglasses. You should also be sure to see an eye specialist if you have had any changes in your vision.

If you smoke, tell your eye doctor. Yes, you will get a lecture, and it is time to listen up if you are still smoking.

Feet: Foot problems are common with diabetes. If your blood glucose has been poorly controlled, you are at risk of developing neuropathy. Because of this nerve damage, you may not be aware of small injuries to your feet. Wound healing may be slowed as well. Small injuries can gradually worsen and become infected.

For this reason, you need to have your doctor check your feet at least once a year. The examination will include a check for sensation using a thin plastic thread, a check of your vibratory sense with a tuning fork, and a thorough check for any signs of damage to your skin. Mary Ellen Wolfe, RN, a nurse who works with George Washington University, also recommends that you take off your shoes and socks at every doctor's visit to be sure your doctor does not forget to examine your feet.

Test Timetable

As directed by your doctor

Blood pressure

Blood glucose levels

CBC

Chemistry panel

Complete foot check (look for injuries, cuts, blisters, etc.)

Every 12 months

Cholesterol levels (total, HDL, LDL, and triglycerides)

Eye exam by an ophthalmologist (to check for retinopathy)

Kidney test (albumin, creatinine, and glomerular filtration rate)

Every 3 to 6 months

Hemoglobin A1c

At each doctor's visit

Blood pressure

Foot exam (visual)

Blood Glucose Testing Cheat Sheet

Know This

The ADA recommends that people with diabetes use the following guidelines for blood glucose levels.

Fasting or before a meal: 90 to 130 mg/dL (5.0 to 7.2 mmol/L)

1 to 2 hours after a meal: lower than 180 mg/dL (10.0 mmol/L)

At bedtime: 100 to 140 mg/dL (5.6 to 7.8 mmol/L)

Do This

If you have type 1 diabetes or are using insulin for type 2 or gestational diabetes, check your glucose at least three times a day or per your doctor's orders.

If you are on oral medication, there is no optimal testing frequency; ask your doctor for a recommendation.

Tell your doctor if you are embarking on a healthier lifestyle such as a diet or exercise program so she can adjust your medication, if necessary.

Carry glucose tablets (which are available at drugstores) with you at all times in case your blood sugar drops too low. (If it goes below 70 mg/dL or whatever number your doctor labels hypoglycemic, you'll need 15 milligrams of glucose right away.)

Wear a medical ID bracelet at all times.

If your blood sugar is developing a pattern of being too high or too low, tell your doctor immediately. Your medication likely needs to be adjusted.

Log This

Track your blood sugar using a logbook or simple chart like this.

BLOOD GLUCOSE READINGS

DATE	MEDICATION REGIMEN	EARLY	BEFORE BREAKFAST	AFTER BREAKFAST	BEFORE LUNCH	AFTER LUNCH	BEFORE DINNER	AFTER DINNER	LATE

Hemoglobin A1c Testing Cheat Sheet ————————

Know This

Your A1c level should be checked every 6 months, or every 3 months if your diet, medications, or general health has changed, or if previous values have been too high.

The ADA says that A1c should be less than 7 percent, and for individual patients for whom further reductions are possible, it should be closer to 6 percent, but this may be difficult to achieve. Ask your doctor to help you set a goal for your A1c levels.

A high A1c level affects your circulation. To keep your heart healthy, also have blood pressure, cholesterol, and other heart tests recommended by your doctor.

Log This

Track your hemoglobin A1c readings using the following chart.

HEMOGLOBIN A1C READINGS

DATE	READING

Be sure to have your A1c level checked at least every 6 months, or every 3 months if your diet, medications, or general health has changed.

Cholesterol Testing Cheat Sheet ───────────

Do This

Make sure your doctor checks your cholesterol levels at least once a year.

Aim for:

Total cholesterol of 150 mg/dL (3.9 mmol/L)

LDL cholesterol of 40 mg/dL (1.0 mmol/L)

HDL cholesterol of above 45 mg/dL (1.2 mmol/L) for men and above 55 mg/dL (1.4 mmol/L) for women

Triglyceride levels of less than 150 mg/dL (3.9 mmol/L)

Log This

Track your cholesterol readings in the following chart.

CHOLESTEROL READINGS

DATE	LDL	HDL	TOTAL	TRIGLYCERIDES

Be sure your doctor checks your cholesterol levels once a year.

Blood Pressure Testing Cheat Sheet

Do This

Aim to keep blood pressure under 130/80 mm Hg. If you have kidney problems or another complication, aim for 125/75 mm Hg. (Normal is 120/80 mm Hg.)

Log This

Track your blood pressure readings using the following chart.

BLOOD PRESSURE READINGS

DATE	READING

Make sure your doctor checks your blood pressure at every visit.

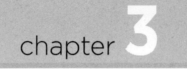
HEALTH CARE HUSBANDING

Save thousands on your health care with these 10 surprising—and easy—ways to trim costs on everything from your yearly physical to specialized surgery

A fter a car accident left Michelle Katz, a Washington, DC, nursing student, with persistent back pain and numbness in 1998, she consulted a neurosurgeon, who told her she'd need an operation to repair her slipped disk. Katz, then 26, didn't have health insurance, so she did the only thing she could think of: She negotiated.

Katz offered to pay her surgeon and anesthesiologist a portion up front in exchange for a hefty discount and arranged a payment plan for the rest. When she got her hospital bill, she haggled with the billing department to drop some charges. All told, she ended up paying just half of the original $28,000 estimate.

"Before this, I didn't think you could negotiate with your doctor," says Katz, 35, now a corporate health care consultant and author of *Healthcare for Less*, which was inspired by her own experience. "But all you have to do is ask."

And ask you should—repeatedly. In 2007, a family of four covered by a typical preferred provider organization (PPO) insurance plan is expected to receive an average of $14,500 in medical services. If you fit that profile, about $5,100 of that will be your responsibility—in the form of premiums, co-pays, and deductibles. That's an increase of more than 8 percent from 2006, following 5 straight years in which costs jumped more than 9 percent annually.

With a little research and some hard bargaining, though, you can cut that figure by half or more. Here are 10 ways to get started, along with the savings you can expect.

SHOP FOR TESTS

Need an expensive test that's going to cost you a hefty out-of-pocket sum? Because fees can vary widely, it might be worthwhile to compare prices among different labs and clinics. To compare prices, you need to know the current procedural terminology (CPT) code, which is a universally accepted number that corresponds to any billable service, such as magnetic resonance imaging (MRI). The American Medical Association's Web site, www.ama-assn.org, has an easy-to-use CPT search engine. Once you have the code, you can get price quotes from several providers. You may be surprised at how well you'll do.

"For a CT scan, the price could range between $500 and $1,500 at two different facilities," says Devon Herrick, PhD, a senior fellow at the National Center for Policy Analysis in Dallas.

Your savings: 20 to 66 percent

NEGOTIATE YOUR HOSPITAL BILL

For patients with insurance, the hospital co-pay or deductible can represent a very large amount of money. Some insurance companies will deduct this amount from the hospital's contracted rate. The unpaid portion is then your responsibility.

Here's a fact many hospitals won't openly admit: They're often willing to waive or reduce an account balance if a patient can demonstrate that the co-pay or deductible is a hardship. But you have to ask.

"The patient can go back to an account administrator and say, 'This is really difficult for me. Is there anything you can do?' And we can," says Ruth Levin, vice president for managed care at Continuum Health Partners in New York City. "The number of payers, including patients and insurance plans, who pay hospitals 100 percent of our charges is probably less than 2 percent."

Your savings: 10 to 30 percent

QUESTION FOLLOW-UP APPOINTMENTS

"When a doctor tells you to come back, whether it's in 3 weeks, 6 months, or a year, ask why. A phone call might suffice," says Arthur Garson Jr., MD, dean and vice president of the University of Virginia School of Medicine and author of *Health Care Half Truths: Too Many Myths, Not Enough Reality.*

When a specialist orders a test, such as an x-ray or MRI, ask your primary care doctor if it's necessary. Seventeen percent of US adults say their doctors have ordered duplicates of medical tests, according to a recent survey by the Commonwealth Fund, which is a non-partisan health care foundation in New York City. If you're going for a second opinion, sign out your x-rays or MRI scans from your doctor and take them with you.

Your savings: $20 (office visit) to $300 (your share of the average cost of an MRI under an insurance plan that reimburses only 80 percent)

No Insurance? Bargain with Cash

If your medical coverage lapses and you need to see a doctor or have a procedure done, offer cash up front. Doctors are often willing to discount their fees in return for guaranteed payment and being able to forgo the hassle of paperwork and administrative costs. Or, offer to match what Medicare would pay—typically about 20 percent less than what a private insurance plan would provide. Medicare reimbursement rates can be found on the American Medical Association's Web site, www.ama-assn.org.

ASK FOR CHEAPER DRUGS

Doctors aren't always aware of how much medication costs. "We don't know which drugs are covered and which aren't when we discuss them with patients," says Doug Farrago, MD, a family physician in Auburn, Maine. Ask your physician if there's a less expensive but equally effective alternative to the drug you're prescribed.

Caveat: "Just be sure your doctor is intimately familiar with the benefits and risks of the alternative drugs for your condition," says Jerome P. Kassirer, MD, distinguished professor at Tufts University School of Medicine in Boston and author of *On the Take: How Medicine's Complicity with Big Business Can Endanger Your Health.*

Your savings: Up to 75 percent (the difference between a "preferred" drug and one not covered by insurance)

PLEAD YOUR CASE DIRECTLY WITH YOUR DOC

If you're experiencing serious hardship, talk directly with your doctor: Doctors are in the profession because they want to do good, so they tend to be more forgiving of outstanding balances than many billing managers are. "They are the ones who can direct their billing department to give the patient a break," says Levin.

Your savings: Up to 70 percent

ARRANGE INDEPENDENT LAB WORK

Cut the cost of blood and urine analyses by using MyMedLab.com. Once your doctor gives you a prescription for a test, have blood drawn at one of 3,000 collection sites nationwide; the vials are then mailed to independent labs.

You can get more than 30 blood readings and analyses starting at about $95, which is around 75 percent less than getting the same tests at a hospital," says Herrick. The lab will mail the results to both you and your doctor. (State laws prohibit this service in California, New Jersey, New York, and Rhode Island, according to the site.)

Caveat: "Ask your doctor to confirm the reliability of an 'outside' lab's performance before using it," says Dr. Kassirer.

Your savings: 50 to 80 percent

HIRE AN ADVOCATE

The gap between what an out-of-network doctor charges for a procedure and what your insurance will pay can often be considerable, and it's usually your responsibility to make up the difference. The result: a three-way dispute. Patient-advocate services are skilled at resolving such conflicts. Philadelphia-based Healthcare Advocates Inc. charges from $50 to $400 per case—about $300 on average.

Caveat: "Ask a representative if he's had success with your particular type of dispute," advises Kassirer. "With some claims, insurance companies never back down." Visit www.prevention.com/advocate to learn how a patient advocate can help you save money.

Your savings: Varies widely

FILL PRESCRIPTIONS WITH BIG RETAILERS

Mail-order pharmacies such as Drugstore.com, Drugs.com, and Costco.com typically beat the prices of neighborhood drugstores hands down. You can do your own price comparisons at Rxaminer.com, which was founded by a cardiologist and has the reputation for independence from special interest groups.

Your savings: 10 to 20 percent for name brands and 20 to 40 percent for generics

SPLIT PILLS

Most drugs are not priced according to strength, points out Fred Brock, a Kansas State University journalism professor and author of *Health Care on Less Than You Think: The* New York Times *Guide to Getting Affordable Coverage*. For example, some popular cholesterol drugs come in at least three strengths. Why not split the 40-milligram pill in half if you need only 20 milligrams per dose, and have the prescription last twice as long? Some pharmacy benefit managers will even give pill splitters to customers at no cost.

Caveat: Splitting pills may not always provide the optimal dose of the drug, so check with your doctor first.

Your savings: Up to 50 percent

E-Shop for the Best Plan

It is possible to price shop for health insurance: Both ehealthinsurance.com and vimo.com offer simple price and coverage comparisons among policies in each state. But never sign up for an insurance plan online. Always talk with a representative before buying, advises Michelle Katz, author of *Healthcare for Less*. "Get their names and numbers so you can go back to them if you have any questions about the information you've seen on the Internet."

TRY BARTERING

"I've had electricians, plumbers, caterers, gardeners, and decorators offer services in exchange for health care," says Dr. Farrago. "If I had a solo practice, I'd do it in a second—though I'm blown away by electricians charging more than I do!"

Caveat: None, "as long as you do a good job for the doctor!" says Dr. Kassirer.

Your savings: Varies widely

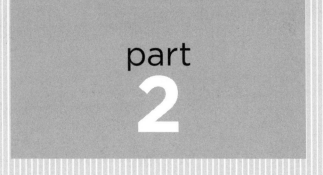

part
2

EAT RIGHT

medical
BREAKTHROUGHS

Want the latest food news? Read on!

EAT THE BREAKFAST OF CHAMPIONS

Go ahead, pour yourself a big bowl: Fiber in cereal, bread, and other grain products may protect against diabetes, according to an *Archives of Internal Medicine* study. Researchers gave more than 25,000 people a food questionnaire and then followed them for 7 years. During that time, 844 of them developed type 2 diabetes.

Researchers found that the people who ate the most cereal fiber (about 17 grams daily) had a 27 percent lower risk of getting diabetes than those who ate the least (about 7 grams). Researchers think that the insoluble fiber in cereal and grains makes cells more sensitive to insulin and that this reduces diabetes risk.

Aim for 25 grams of fiber a day, and get your quota from whole-grain breads, cereals, and health bars such as Gnu Foods Flavor & Fiber bars.

Another study, this one by University of Toronto scientists, found that when 77 people munched on various cereals, blood tests revealed that those with insulin resistance had elevated blood sugar and insulin levels after eating low-fiber cereal, but they had normal levels when they ate high-fiber cereal (3 to 5 grams per bowl).

Pour on fat-free or 1 percent milk for extra protection: Research suggests that a daily serving can slash insulin resistance risk by 20 percent, thanks to its vitamin D.

"A healthy high-fiber breakfast could cut your risk for insulin resistance by 30 to 50 percent," says JoAnne Rizzotto, RD, a nutritionist at the Joslin Diabetes Center in Boston. "If you need something sweet, add some berries to your high-fiber cereal."

BE LOW WITH BARLEY

Eat barley for breakfast, and the rest of your meals will be less fattening, states a new Swedish study. When 20 adults ate barley in the morning, the grain cut their blood sugar response by 44 percent at lunch and 14 percent at dinner.

And the less your sugar spikes, the less fat your body will store. Credit the high amount of soluble fiber in barley, which takes hours to digest. Plus, according to the study authors, the fiber's effect on glucose remains active while it breaks down.

Opt for high-barley bread or pick up pearl barley at www.homegrownharvest.com ($3.50 for 2 pounds). Mix the cooked grain into yogurt or oatmeal.

As a bonus, barley also lowers low-density lipoprotein (LDL) cholesterol (the "bad" cholesterol) levels.

BAR THE MUNCHIES

Energy bars are just the ticket for a quick snack on the go. But many of them seem like glorified (and expensive!) candy bars that actually slow you down instead of pepping you up.

With some smart sleuthing, though, you can find energy bars with a low glycemic index rating that will both rev up your energy and turn down your appetite. Lower-glycemic-index foods send fewer simple sugars into your bloodstream, generating smaller blood sugar (glucose) swings and delaying hunger longer.

Researchers at Pennsylvania State University analyzed three top-selling bars. The lower the glycemic index rating, the better the appetite suppression. Here's how they stack up.

Sugar water (for comparison): glycemic index rating of 100

Slim-Fast Meal Options Optima rich chocolate brownie bar: glycemic index rating of 63.8

Zone Perfect double chocolate nutrition bar: glycemic index rating of 43.7

Best bet: Hershey's SmartZone chocolate nutrition bar: glycemic index rating of 10.9

BURN SLOWER

Carb junkies, rejoice! Purdue University researchers have found a way to change the structure of cornstarch so it takes longer to digest and releases less sugar. The result: less of the blood sugar spike that's normally triggered by eating baked goods or foods cooked in cornstarch-thickened sauces and gravies. That spike—and the crash that follows—causes us to feel hungry soon after eating. Next up: testing the new cornstarch on humans to see whether they down fewer muffins.

CASH IN YOUR CHIPS

Shovel your salsa with a bag of blues: Blue tortillas pack a healthier punch than white ones, reports a study in the *Journal of the Science of Food and Agriculture*. The colorful crisps contain nearly 20 percent more protein and 10 percent less starch. The starch they do contain is of the slowly digested variety.

This keeps blood sugar levels from roller-coastering, which helps combat obesity and insulin resistance, says lead researcher Juscelino Tovar, PhD. Plus, the tint comes from anthocyanins—the same antioxidants responsible for the disease-fighting power of blueberries and red wine.

SOY YES

Soy protein isn't one of the building blocks of the typical American diet, but perhaps it should be, especially for people with diabetes. Researchers in Iran followed 41 people with diabetes for 4 years. They divided the people into two groups.

The first group ate a diet of 35 percent animal protein (such as chicken), 35 percent textured soy protein (such as tofu), and 30 percent vegetable protein (such as beans). The second group ate a diet sans soy, of 70 percent animal protein and 30 percent vegetable protein. Both groups received the same medical treatments for their diabetes.

The researchers discovered that the people who ate the soy protein had significantly lower levels of blood sugar, total cholesterol, LDL cholesterol, and triglycerides.

"Based on these findings, people with diabetes should talk with their doctors or nutritionists about incorporating soy into their diets, such as a serving of tofu a day," says study author Leila Azadbakht, PhD.

NO YOKING

The incredible, edible, *deadly* egg? Nutrition research has been contradictory about whether eggs are nature's most perfect food or are unsafe to eat. A recent study by researchers at Brigham and Women's Hospital and Harvard Medical School, both in Boston, is firmly in the "unsafe" camp.

Researchers studied more than 21,000 men as part of the larger Physicians' Health Study and found that although men without diabetes could eat up to six eggs a week without increasing their risk of death, men with diabetes who ate five or more eggs per week had a two-fold increased risk of death over diabetic men who did not consume eggs. The study suggested that eating eggs may have caused a greater risk for strokes and heart attack among people with diabetes. However, this study did not have enough cases of heart attacks and strokes among diabetic men to provide a definitive answer. Researchers do not know yet whether such findings will be observed in women.

The study authors aren't sure why eggs could be hazardous to the health of people with diabetes. Perhaps it's because they are high in cholesterol, which in high amounts can clog arteries and raise the risk of stroke and heart attack.

"Current studies are suggesting that frequent consumption of eggs may carry additional risk for cardiovascular disease, especially among people with diabetes, and it may be prudent to limit egg consumption to less than 5 per week," says study author Luc Djoussé, MD. "Because new studies may further clarify the link between eggs and cardiovascular disease in people with diabetes, it is always a good idea to check with your doctor whenever you have concerns."

CIN A LITTLE

Like Lindsay Lohan in *Mean Girls*, cinnamon is a good kid that got mixed up with a bad crowd. The fatty results: cinnamon buns, cinnamon sugar, cinnamon swirl raisin bread. But without the sugar, cinnamon's effect on your health is better than good—it's fantastic.

"It's emerging as a true wonder food in terms of health protection," says Ann Kulze, MD, a physician in Mount Pleasant, South Carolina, and author of *Dr. Ann's 10-Step Diet.*

Research has linked the copper-colored stuff with reduced blood sugar, cholesterol, and triglyceride levels in people with type 2 diabetes, and a recent study published in the *American Journal of Clinical Nutrition* found that adding a little more than a teaspoon to rice pudding even helped tame blood sugar in people without diabetes. Dr. Kulze says cinnamon also contains polyphenols, which are antioxidants that create healthier arteries and reduce the risk of cardiovascular disease. The spice's energizing scent has also been found to help increase alertness.

But that isn't even the best part: Cinnamon is easy to add to food you already eat and makes everything taste better. Both ground and stick forms are equally healthy, but sticks have a longer shelf life (1 year, compared with 6 months for ground). There's no need to grind your own: Preground store-bought is as good as fresh ground and saves the hassle. Aim for ½ to 1½ teaspoons (or one to two sticks) a day, Dr. Kulze recommends. Try the following tricks to get more of the nice spice.

Add ½ to 1½ teaspoons to hot oatmeal or cold cereal.

Add 1 tablespoon to pancake batter.

Mix ½ teaspoon into 2 tablespoons of peanut butter and spread onto celery sticks.

Microwave 1 cup of soy milk and 1 teaspoon of honey for 1 minute and 30 seconds, then add ½ teaspoon. Or simmer a stick and honey in soy milk for 5 minutes on the stove.

Stir ½ teaspoon into plain yogurt.

Sprinkle $\frac{1}{2}$ teaspoon over sweet potatoes or carrots.

Toss $\frac{1}{4}$ to $\frac{1}{2}$ teaspoon over broiled grapefruit or bananas.

Add 2 teaspoons to a store-bought rub for grilled chicken or pork.

Coat 2 cups of raw nuts with a mix of $\frac{1}{4}$ cup of honey and $\frac{1}{2}$ teaspoon of cinnamon, and roast at 350°F for 15 minutes.

Shake three dashes into your favorite fruit smoothie.

Sprinkle $\frac{1}{2}$ teaspoon straight into your coffee, latte, or cappuccino.

SPICE IT UP

Don't leave the supplement aisle without picking up some fenugreek seed extract. Never heard of it? You're in good company, but here's why you need to give it a look.

In a small study in India, people with type 2 diabetes who took 1 gram of fenugreek seed extract for 2 months reduced blood sugar levels by about 20 percent, the same amount as those who followed a standard nutrition and exercise program.

"It's safe for most people," says Ryan Bradley, ND, head of the Diabetes and Cardio-vascular Wellness Program at Bastyr University. (Follow label instructions; do *not* take fenugreek if you're on blood thinners.)

Fenugreek may be a helpful addition to your diabetes treatment plan, but talk with your doctor before trying this or any other type of supplement. And make sure you continue managing your condition with medication, activity, and a healthy diet.

STABILIZE WITH YERBA MATÉ

Maté (MAH-tay), a plant native to Argentina and used to make a tealike infusion, has an herbal taste and half the caffeine of coffee.

It's like green tea on steroids, with up to 90 percent more powerful cancer-fighting anti-oxidants, a cache of B vitamins, and plenty of chromium, which helps stabilize blood sugar levels. Plus, its bolstering effect on metabolism is so valued that many diet pills list maté as an ingredient.

For the strongest dose of maté's medicine, buy loose-leaf bags at www.guayaki.com. Or find flavored varieties from Bombilla Gourd at your local Whole Foods store. Be sure to talk with your doctor before giving it a try, however.

BAG SUGAR SPIKES

Black tea reduces the glycemic index of a meal, according to a new study in the *Journal of the American College of Nutrition*. When British researchers had twelve people drink 12 ounces of the hot beverage after eating a high-carbohydrate meal, the participants' sugar levels decreased 40 percent more in just 2 hours than did the levels of those who didn't drink tea.

"An active compound in the tea triggers a greater secretion of insulin, a hormone that lowers blood sugar," says the study's coauthor, Peter Ellis, PhD.

RAISE A GLASS

White wine goes great with carbohydrates. When Australian scientists served adults an alcoholic drink with a high-carbohydrate dinner, they observed that the drink significantly reduced the glycemic index of the meal. As a result, the study participants' blood sugar levels didn't rise as much after the meal as when they downed water instead.

The benefit? "Keeping your blood sugar in check can help prevent chronic diseases, such as diabetes and heart disease," says study author Jennie Brand-Miller, PhD. Compared with beer and gin, white wine has the greatest effect, lowering the meal's glycemic index by 37 percent. "The high acidity of white wine may help slow digestion, keeping sugar from entering your bloodstream as quickly," Brand-Miller says.

Keep this in mind, however, when knocking one back: Drinking alcohol can lead to low blood sugar in some people with diabetes. This is especially true if you're on a medication such as insulin or certain pills that can cause low blood glucose.

For most people with diabetes, however, the occasional drink is probably okay (although it's a great idea to check with your doctor to be sure). But don't drink on an empty stomach: Have a carbohydrate snack such as whole-grain crackers, or enjoy your drink with a meal. The American Diabetes Association (ADA) suggests that women with diabetes have no more than one drink a day and that men with diabetes have no more than two.

Remember, too, that alcohol packs calories, which can pack on the pounds. One drink—which is 4 ounces of wine, 12 ounces of beer, or 1 ounce of hard liquor—contains approximately 80 to 150 calories.

POP GOES YOUR HEALTH

Regularly drinking just half a can of soda raises your risk of diabetes. When Finnish researchers tracked the diets of 4,000 adults for more than a decade, they found that people who drink 6 ounces of soda daily are 67 percent more likely to have type 2 diabetes than are nonsoda drinkers. How can such a small amount wreak so much havoc? The researchers aren't sure, but they do know this: "People who consume these beverages have poor diets in general," says study author Jukka Montonen, PhD. In fact, Purdue University scientists recently concluded that sugar-free-soda drinkers make healthier nutritional choices than those who sip the sugar-laden kind.

chapter 4

THE GOOD CARBS

Try this amazing Rx for diabetes

The glycemic index (sometimes abbreviated "GI") system for rating carbs may help you beat diabetes, heart attacks, an appetite that's out of control, and more. And it may offer dramatic health benefits not just for people with diabetes but for almost everyone.

Invented in the early 1980s by University of Toronto researchers as a tool to help control diabetes, the glycemic index ranks carbohydrate foods by their effect on your blood sugar levels.

"We're learning that the type of carbs you eat really makes a difference in your health," says glycemic index researcher Christine L. Pelkman, PhD, of Pennsylvania State University in State College. And the glycemic index helps you choose the best carbs for you. You can use the glycemic index to choose meals and snacks that give you an edge against diabetes, heart attacks, and possibly even cancer. And don't be surprised if you find yourself losing weight to boot. For a list of common foods, visit Prevention.com and search on "Your Guide to the Glycemic Index."

GOOD CARBS, NOT-SO-GOOD CARBS

The glycemic index assigns foods containing carbs a number based on how they affect your blood sugar, or blood glucose, after you eat them. Foods with a glycemic index of less than 55 cause only a little blip in blood sugar; those in the 55 to 70 range raise it a little higher; and carbs with a glycemic index of more than 70 send blood sugar soaring. Low-glycemic-index carbs are healthy; high-glycemic-index carbs, in excess, are not.

What explains the difference in numbers? No matter what form the carbs initially take—the lactose in milk, the starch in a bagel, the sucrose in table sugar—eventually, your body breaks it down to glucose. Glucose winds up in your bloodstream, fueling your cells. What makes a glycemic index number high or low is how quickly the food breaks down during digestion. The longer your body has to wrestle with the carbs to break them down into glucose, the slower the rise in blood sugar and the lower the glycemic index.

But it's not always easy to predict a food's glycemic index. Often, fiber-rich foods have lower glycemic indexes. Fiber, especially the soluble type in oats and beans, creates a web in the intestines that traps carb particles. Not surprisingly, beans have low-glycemic-index numbers. But when fiber is ground finely, as it often is in whole wheat flour, it doesn't present enough of a digestive challenge to lower the glycemic index of these foods. That explains why whole wheat bread has a glycemic index number nearly identical to that of white bread. (But whole wheat bread is still a healthier choice than white bread is, because of its extra fiber and other nutrients.)

Surprisingly, table sugar has a lower glycemic index than potatoes do. That's because it's made of two sugars, glucose and fructose; the glucose half sails right into the bloodstream, but the fructose segment has to detour through the liver, where it slowly gets converted into glucose. But the starch molecules in potatoes are strings of glucose. Boiling, baking, or mashing a potato causes the starch molecules to burst, making it easy for glucose to enter the bloodstream.

HIGH GLYCEMIC INDEX = HIGH RISK

The problem with eating lots of high-glycemic-index foods is this: When your blood sugar soars, so does the hormone insulin. Insulin's main duty is to scoop up excess blood sugar and store it safely in muscle tissue. In moderation, insulin is a good guy, but it becomes a killer when its levels spike repeatedly, triggering diabetes, heart disease, and possibly cancer. Unfortunately, insulin is spiking all the time in the millions of Americans who consume high-glycemic-index fare such as bagels, doughnuts, french fries, and other quickly absorbed starchy carbohydrates. Experts point out that modern diets offer vastly more opportunity to eat starchy high-glycemic-index foods than did the diets on which human beings evolved.

TAMING THE KILLERS

The good news is that switching to a low-glycemic-index diet results in a minimum outpouring of insulin, and that has healthy ramifications all over your body. Here's what a low-glycemic-index diet appears to help you do.

Stop diabetes. Diabetes, characterized by above-normal blood sugar, has reached epidemic proportions in the United States, afflicting almost 21 million Americans. Most have type 2 diabetes, prompted by two very American conditions: excess weight and a sedentary lifestyle. And millions more are walking around with a degree of insulin resistance just shy of diabetes.

"The beauty of the glycemic index for diabetics is that it not only helps control blood sugar and insulin, but its appetite-suppressing effects help them lose weight. And weight loss alone can reverse type 2 diabetes," says Marc Rendell, MD, director of the Creighton Diabetes Center at Creighton University in Omaha, Nebraska, and medical director of the Rose Salter Medical Research Foundation in Baltimore. Although Dr. Rendell believes that it's entirely possible to induce remission of many cases of type 2 diabetes by using the glycemic index, he urges patients with diabetes to continue their current therapies and to add only low-glycemic-index foods in consultation with a physician or registered dietitian.

Research testing low- versus high-glycemic-index diets for people with diabetes is promising. A 1999 Swedish study of people with type 2 diabetes found that 4 weeks on a low-glycemic-index diet lowered blood glucose and insulin by 30 percent compared with a high-glycemic-index diet. In a 4-month study led by the University of Toronto's Thomas Wolever, MD, a low-glycemic-index diet markedly improved insulin sensitivity in a group of prediabetic insulin-resistant people. "If these trends were sustained, these people could probably avoid getting diabetes," Dr. Wolever says.

This is exactly the implication of several large-scale diet surveys. In a 6-year study of male health professionals, men eating the lowest-glycemic-index diets were 25 percent less likely to get diabetes. In the Nurses' Health Study, the most powerful diabetes protection—a drop in risk of one-third or more—came from eating a low-glycemic-index diet and getting lots of fiber from cereal (7.5 grams daily).

Drop pounds. Ever feel hungry just an hour or two after a meal? It could be because the meal had a high glycemic index. Ironically, high-glycemic-index meals cause such a flood of insulin, for coping with all the glucose, that blood sugar levels wind up lower than if you'd never eaten. And low blood sugar may send out hunger alarms, according to Susan Roberts, PhD, professor of nutrition at Tufts University in Boston and author of *Feeding Your Child for Lifelong Health.* In one study, overweight children (average age 10) at Children's Hospital in Boston spent 4 months on either a low-glycemic-index diet or a low-fat diet of equal calories. The clear winner: the low-glycemic-index diet, with an average weight loss of 4.5 pounds compared with 2.8 pounds on the low-fat diet.

Roberts suspects that high-glycemic-index carbs are partly behind America's epidemic levels of obesity. "GI is not the complete answer to everyone's weight problem. But aside from the research, I am personally convinced that low-GI diets help people lose weight, myself included. My husband and I were eating either a relatively high-GI instant oatmeal or a low-GI Irish oatmeal for breakfast, and I'd call and ask how he felt 2 hours later. Both of us noticed a big decrease in hunger with the low-GI oatmeal. Now I've become very aware of the GI of what I eat and quite consistently find myself hungrier after very high-GI foods such as bagels, mashed potatoes, and the like."

Keep your heart strong. High levels of insulin wreak havoc on the heart. "Elevated insulin triggers a bevy of heart disease risk factors," says Michael Zemel, PhD, chairman of the department of nutrition at the University of Tennessee in Knoxville. Zemel reviewed the connections between glycemic index and heart disease and found that they include high blood pressure, increased fat storage, high triglycerides (a type of blood fat), and lower levels of high-density lipoprotein (HDL) (the "good" cholesterol). Once again, low-glycemic-index foods appear to be the Rx. In the Nurses' Health Study, women eating diets with the most carbohydrates from high-glycemic-index foods were nearly twice as likely to develop heart disease.

Thwart cancer: A high-glycemic-index diet may even be linked to colon cancer. The hypothesis: The flood of insulin, glucose, and blood fats that stem from a high-glycemic-index diet fuel colon cancer cells. Both human and animal research support this theory. For instance, colon cancer patients are prone to insulin resistance, and giving insulin speeds up the development of colon cancer in rats.

Stay energetic and alert: Want more stamina? You have greater endurance when you exercise after a low-glycemic-index meal than after a high-glycemic-index meal, most studies show. And low-glycemic-index meals might also give you a mental edge, hints Australian research. People who ate a low-glycemic-index breakfast scored higher in a test of alertness than did those who ate a high-glycemic-index breakfast.

"I think the low-GI breakfast increased alertness for two reasons: by fueling the brain with a slow, steady supply of glucose and by staving off hunger," says study leader Susanna Holt, PhD, RD, of Sydney University's Human Nutrition Unit. "People eating this breakfast didn't get hungry before lunch, while those eating corn flakes did. It's easier to be alert and focused when you're not hungry."

Although organizations in other countries, such as the Canadian Diabetes Association, Australia's International Diabetes Institute, and the World Health Organization, all recommend including low-glycemic-index foods as part of managing diabetes, the glycemic index gets only a brief mention in practice guidelines from the American Diabetes Association (ADA). "At this point, we don't recommend the glycemic index because not enough is known, and there's no evidence that this method is better than the standard approach of counting carbohydrates," says Marian Parrot, MD, vice president of clinical affairs for the ADA. Although Dr. Parrot agrees that the glycemic index is "not harmful" and that "nothing is wrong with the science," her main objection is that it's too complicated. People just can't be expected to remember and deal with all those numbers. And in fact, a substantial group of health experts agrees that although the glycemic index may prove useful someday, it is "not ready for prime time." But in response, Creighton Diabetes Center's Dr. Rendell, who wrote a 2000 editorial backing the glycemic index in the prestigious *New England Journal of Medicine*, believes there's a bias against publishing research in this area. "It's just

Peruse the Pasta Aisle

Lately, pasta has been getting a pretty bad rap. Critics contend that regular pasta is as nutritious as the box it's sold in, and that whole wheat pasta tastes about as good as that cardboard does. But that is about to change, because whole-grain pasta is now better tasting—and better for you!—than ever.

Here's why: Whole grains retain all the disease-fighting, health-promoting powerhouse nutrients that get stripped away in the refining process (such as folate, vitamin E, magnesium, potassium, selenium, lignans, and phenolic compounds). They also pack more fiber than refined grains do, and large studies have repeatedly shown that consuming enough fiber can help reduce your risk of heart disease and diabetes. Oh, and yes, eating whole grains may even help you avoid weight gain.

Look a little closer at the pasta aisle these days. You'll likely find close to a dozen different brands of whole-grain pasta, maybe even more than regular pasta. The choices run the gamut between pure 100 percent whole wheat (which contains no refined flour) and grain blends (which don't always have as much fiber but make up for it with more-pleasant textures and less assertive flavors). The latest blends combine various grain flours with seeds, legumes, and other ingredients to improve the texture while preserving nutrition. Some offer nutrients you aren't likely to find in traditional pasta, such as omega-3 fatty acids (thanks to flax). Here are three of the very best.

not politically correct. I've seen excellent research papers on the GI get put aside by medical journals; unfortunately, the best studies haven't been published," he asserts.

"The authorities in the field are too hung up on arithmetic," he says. "For instance, they bring up the fact that carrots have a high GI, so they're afraid people will stop eating carrots." But glycemic index experts never advise avoiding high-glycemic-index foods that are low-calorie salad vegetables or fruits. "If high-GI foods such as carrots are also low in calories, you'd have to eat pounds of them to make much of an impact on blood

Highest Fiber: De Cecco Whole Wheat

100 percent whole wheat.

High in fiber, low in calories.

Fairly assertive wheat flavor that marries well with rich sauces.

Per serving: 180 cal, 8 g pro, 35 g carb, 1.5 g fat, 0 g sat fat, <5 mg chol, 7 g fiber, 0 mg sodium

Bonus Nutrients: Barilla Plus

A multigrain blend made with oat, spelt, barley, lentil, and chickpea flours.

Contains flaxseed for added omega-3s.

Each serving satisfies nearly one-fifth of your daily value for protein.

Taste and texture are like refined-flour pasta.

Per serving: 200 cal, 10 g pro, 38 g carb, 1 g fat, 0 g sat fat, 0 mg chol, 4 g fiber, 25 mg sodium

Tasty Blend: Ronzoni Healthy Harvest

Wheat flour blend with additional wheat bran and fiber.

Slightly chewier and nuttier in flavor than Barilla Plus.

Best served with robust sauces, such as marinara.

Per serving: 180 cal, 6 g pro, 42 g carb, 1 g fat, 0 g sat fat, 0 mg chol, 6 g fiber, 0 mg sodium

sugar," says the University of Toronto's Dr. Wolever, coauthor of *The Glucose Revolution*. He recommends targeting those high-glycemic-index foods that are also high in calories, such as baked goods, highly refined breakfast cereals, and potatoes. Start to replace them with lower-glycemic-index foods, such as trading in bagels for 100 percent stone-ground whole wheat bread, instant rice for barley, or corn flakes for All-Bran. "Switching to these low-GI starches," says Dr. Wolever, "can make a tremendous difference in your health."

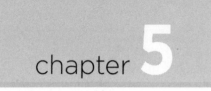

chapter 5

GROCERY CART MAKEOVERS

Join our nutritionist as she shows three women what to skip and what to pick in every aisle

Y
ou enter the grocery store with the best of intentions: to buy healthy foods for yourself and your family. But it's easy to go through on autopilot—buying the same things over and over, even when you suspect (or know) that your choices aren't good for you. To the rescue: strategic shopping—zoning in on the exact foods you need for meeting your biggest nutrition goal.

We asked expert Tanya Zuckerbrot, RD, author of the fiber-based weight loss book *The F-Factor Diet*, to guide three women through the supermarket to show us how it should be done. What they learned can make reaching your own healthy eating goals easy.

GOAL: GET HEALTHY PREPREGNANCY

Lisa Perkins, age 43, obstacle: a preference for high-fat foods

Although Lisa buys plenty of fruits and veggies, her cart has too many saturated fat–filled dairy products and meats, such as cottage cheese and sausage. Switching just a few to lower-fat versions will help her maintain a healthy weight. She'd also benefit from better carb choices. The white bread and corn flakes she eats are too low in fiber and high in sugar.

Her New Strategy

Seek folate-rich greens. Adequate folate intake will help prevent birth defects, should Lisa get pregnant. The best sources are dark-green leafy vegetables such as spinach and Brussels sprouts (frozen is fine, too), and she should try to eat some every day.

Choose fiber-rich cereal. Fiber One, Kashi GoLean, or any type of cereal with 5 grams or more of fiber per serving is a good choice. "By slowly incorporating fiber into her diet to reach the recommended 25 grams a day, she will help reduce the likelihood of pregnancy-related problems, such as hemorrhoids and gestational diabetes, later," says Zuckerbrot.

Look for low-fat dairy. Whole milk has 8 grams of fat per serving; Lisa has several servings a day. "When I told her to choose products labeled low fat, she grimaced," says Zuckerbrot. "She doesn't always have to choose the light version; even once in a while would be an improvement." Low-fat milk has all the nutrients of whole, and low-fat American, goat, and ricotta cheeses taste as good as their regular versions. To help Lisa make the switch from thick-and-creamy-style yogurt, Zuckerbrot suggested low-fat Greek-style yogurt, which is strained so it has a thicker texture, without the extra fat and sugar.

Try healthier bacon. "Lisa didn't want to drop bacon from her diet, but she was willing to compromise," says Zuckerbrot. "I told her to save the regular kind for special occasions, and buy bacon labeled reduced fat, Canadian bacon, or turkey bacon the rest of the time." For each slice of turkey bacon she swaps in, she saves 1 gram of fat and at least 12 calories.

Did It Help?

"I loved that the suggestions were doable," Lisa says. "Switching to turkey bacon was pretty painless; my boyfriend and I had already tried it, so now we just eat it more often. I'm not yet convinced on the low-fat cottage cheese—the texture doesn't seem right to me—but I've resolved to buy lower-fat yogurt and high-fiber cereal the next time I go shopping."

"I thought I was being healthy by choosing ground turkey, but because it contains dark meat, it has as much fat and calories as beef. The fix was easy, though: Look for ground turkey labeled extra-lean that has no more than 4 grams of fat in a serving."

GOAL: FAST, HEALTHY MEALS

Jeanne Achille, age 51, obstacle: a finicky family

Like most moms with hectic schedules, Jeanne needs dishes she can throw together in 5 minutes. What she doesn't realize is that fast food can be healthy, if you make the right choices. The boxed macaroni and cheese she buys is too high in calories, but her bagged salads and ready-made sushi combos are better. What makes shopping especially hard for Jeanne is that she has many different palates to please: Her 17-year-old avoids carbs, but her husband loves them. The key is finding a happy medium, which, for her family, are meals with high-fiber carbs and protein.

Her New Strategy

Make to-go meals healthier. For lunch, Jeanne often heads to the hot food bar for fried chicken and rice. And she makes her way back for dinner, which is either ready-made pasta or Chinese noodles. Sometimes it's a frozen Thai chicken dish from the freezer section, which is loaded with fat and sodium and contains virtually no fiber.

Zuckerbrot reroutes Jeanne to the deli counter for both meals. Sliced turkey on whole wheat has only about 225 calories; her frozen dish has 500. And a precooked rotisserie chicken makes an easy dinner for three. Just remove the skin and pair it with a deli salad tossed in a light vinaigrette, such as asparagus salad or carrot-and-raisin slaw. Or shred the chicken with a fork and mix with a few tablespoons of barbecue sauce. This is "kind of like pulled pork but with healthier chicken," says Zuckerbrot.

Pick precut and no-cut veggies. Peeled baby carrots, cherry tomatoes, and hearts of celery are easy additions to prewashed salad greens. Frozen and canned vegetables are good for omelets, pasta sauce, or a stir-fry—all meals that take about 10 minutes to cook. "You really have no excuse not to eat veggies," says Zuckerbrot. "All the work is done for you."

Do a carb swap. "You can eat carbs and lose weight," says Zuckerbrot. "What's important is the quantity and the quality." Stick to the recommended portion sizes and trade processed breads, pastas, English muffins, and tortillas for whole-grain versions. They offer additional nutrients. "If her hubby objects to whole wheat pasta, she can opt for a blend of white and wheat, such as Barilla Plus," says Zuckerbrot. For a fast and delicious pasta dinner, blend mixed-wheat pasta with low-fat cheese, or add some tomato sauce and part-skim ricotta.

Go dark with chocolate. "The darker, the better," says Zuckerbrot. "It contains more antioxidants." Jeanne, who eats chocolate every day, might try Hershey's Kisses Special Dark. Zuckerbrot likes its built-in portion control, which is perfect for when those too-big chocolate candy bars call Jeanne's name.

Did It Help?

"Tanya showed me that all I had to do was swap a few foods on my shopping list for their healthier versions," Jeanne says. "Frozen veggie burgers are my new fast, favorite meal, and instead of frozen broccoli and cheese as a side dish, I pick up Birds Eye Steamfresh frozen broccoli or cut green beans. I love that I can cook them in the microwave in just a few minutes, without even removing them from the bag. My husband did raise his eyebrows at the idea of switching from regular to whole wheat pasta, but we're working on it. And while I was a little skeptical that one dark chocolate kiss would curb my cravings, it really worked!"

"I had no idea the cream-based salad dressings I always used had 16 grams of fat and more than 150 calories per serving. Now I spray greens with olive oil (to help me control how much I use), drizzle with balsamic vinegar (thicker because it's aged), and top with a little grated Parmesan for extra flavor."

GOAL: LOSE 10 POUNDS

Karen Quinn, age 51, obstacle: her two teenagers who love junk food

Karen's cart was loaded with processed and refined foods such as corn chips, brownies, and white bread, and it was way too light on fruits and vegetables. Zuckerbrot was happy to see fat-free milk (she needs the calcium to keep her bones strong), but the "diet" snacks she favors, such as reduced-sugar chocolate chip cookies, won't satisfy her sweet tooth—and will end up doing her diet more harm than good.

Her New Strategy

Head straight to produce. "This should be stop number one if you want to lose weight," says Zuckerbrot. "Fruits and vegetables fill you up with few calories." It took a little digging, but eventually, this veggie avoider conceded she didn't mind salad greens, avocados, mushrooms, apples, and berries—so that's exactly what she should buy and add to her diet any way she can—in omelets, as snacks, or grilled as a side dish. "But go easy on high-cal avocados," advises Zuckerbrot. "One-eighth—or two slices—is a serving."

Trim fat at the meat counter. "Pass on rib eyes and pick up much-leaner tenderloin fillets or flank steak," suggests Zuckerbrot. Karen's kids love chicken made with Shake 'n Bake; if she removes the skin before cooking, she'll save more than 4 grams of fat and about 50 calories.

Trade white for wheat. Karen's son won't go near whole wheat bread, so she should try Wonder's version, which looks white but is actually whole grain, says Zuckerbrot. "Kids won't know the difference." The whole grain is healthier, and the fiber will help Karen feel fuller longer. Whatever brand you buy, check the label: "Avoid those with more than 15 to 20 grams of sugar or 200 calories per serving," says Zuckerbrot.

Skip "diet" snacks. Karen hadn't bought regular peanut butter in 20 years, but the fat in it is actually heart healthy. Because her family likes desserts, Karen buys the low-fat versions for herself, but their less-satisfying texture and taste may encourage munching. She may have more success curbing cravings with fruit or small portions of the real thing (such as one fresh bakery cookie).

Did It Help?

"This was a life-changing experience," Karen says. "Tanya not only helped me rethink my food choices but also figured out how many calories I should eat daily to lose weight (about 1,200). Admittedly, her tip to eat berries with a little Splenda and lemon juice didn't go over well with my daughter. She thought it tasted funny. But I made my son a sandwich

Your Four-Step Strategic Shopping Plan

Whatever your diet goal—be it weight loss, having more energy, eating more nutrients, or keeping your heart healthy—follow these tips from Tanya Zuckerbrot, RD.

Fuel up before you go. Hunger is the number one reason women buy food they know they shouldn't. Have a 100- to 200-calorie snack containing some fat, protein, and carbohydrates about 30 minutes before you hit the store. A good choice is crackers with peanut butter and a piece of fruit.

Load good foods first. The initial items you put into your shopping cart should be those that meet your main dietary goals. That way, if you run out of time or get impatient and leave quickly, you'll already have what you need most in your cart and be ready for checkout. For example, if your goal is fast, healthy dinners, pick up the ingredients for a stir-fry before moving on to cereals.

Always do a quick label check. Taking 5 seconds to read the nutrition information can save you hundreds of calories and dozens of grams of fat. Even if you've purchased an item in the past, ingredients change, so it never hurts to look.

Shop for snacks last. If your cart is full, you'll be less likely to buy a half-dozen varieties. And look for portion-controlled snacks in 100-calorie packs. They cost a bit more, but the calories you'll save are worth every penny.

---

with whole-grain 'white' bread, and he ate it without saying a word! I now eat high-fiber cereal with berries and fat-free milk for breakfast, and I'm barely hungry by the time lunch rolls around!"

"When Tanya told me frozen fries are full of fat, my jaw hit the floor. I didn't realize they were fried in oil and then frozen! Now I make my own: Slice up a regular potato, coat with cooking spray, and bake. I save up to 100 calories and more than 6 grams of fat."

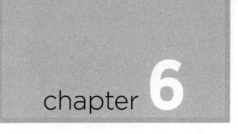

chapter 6

THE GREAT EIGHT

Eat these fabulous foods every day

I t sometimes seems as if the internal politics of Baghdad are easier to sort through than the latest thinking on nutrition. So here's the simple solution: Just eat these eight foods—along with a little protein such as salmon, turkey, or lean steak—every day. And relax. Let our all-star panel of doctors, scientists, nutritionists, and chefs tell you why and show you how.

SPINACH

What it's great for: sexual enhancement, muscle growth, heart health, bone strength, eyesight

Men, in particular, take note on this one! Spinach may be green and leafy, but it is also the ultimate man food. This noted biceps builder is a rich source of plant-based omega-3s and folate, which help reduce the risk of heart disease, stroke, and osteoporosis. Bonus: Folate also increases blood flow to the penis. And spinach is packed with lutein, which is a compound that fights age-related macular degeneration.

Aim for: 1 cup of fresh spinach or ½ cup cooked per day.

Substitutes: Kale, bok choy, and romaine lettuce

Fit it in: Make your salads with spinach; add spinach to scrambled eggs; drape it over pizza; mix it with marinara sauce and then microwave for an instant dip.

Pinch hitter: Sesame Stir-Braised Kale: Heat 4 cloves of minced garlic, 1 tablespoon of minced fresh ginger, and 1 teaspoon of sesame oil in a skillet. Add 2 tablespoons of water and 1 bunch of kale (stemmed and chopped). Cover and cook for 3 minutes. Drain. Add 1 teaspoon of soy sauce and 1 tablespoon of sesame seeds.

YOGURT

What it's great for: fighting cancer, bone strength, boosting immunity

Various cultures claim yogurt as their own creation, but the 2,000-year-old food's health benefits are not disputed: Fermentation spawns hundreds of millions of probiotic organisms that serve as reinforcements to the battalions of beneficial bacteria in your body, which boost the immune system and provide protection against cancer. Not all yogurts are probiotic though, so make sure the label says "live and active cultures."

Aim for: 1 cup of the calcium- and protein-rich goop a day.

Substitutes: Kefir, soy yogurt

Fit it in: Yogurt topped with blueberries, walnuts, flaxseed, and honey is the ultimate breakfast—or dessert. Plain low-fat yogurt is also a perfect base for creamy salad dressings and dips.

Home run: Power Smoothie: Blend 1 cup of low-fat yogurt, 1 cup of fresh or frozen blueberries, 1 cup of carrot juice, and 1 cup of fresh baby spinach for a nutrient-rich blast.

TOMATOES

What they're great for: cancer fighting, heart health, immunity boosting

There are two things you need to know about tomatoes: Red are the best, because they're packed with more of the antioxidant lycopene, and processed tomatoes are just as potent as fresh ones, because it's easier for the body to absorb the lycopene. Studies show that a diet rich in lycopene can decrease your risk of bladder, lung, prostate, skin, and stomach cancers, as well as reduce the risk of coronary artery disease.

Aim for: 22 milligrams of lycopene a day, which is about eight red cherry tomatoes or a glass of tomato juice.

Substitutes: Red watermelon, pink grapefruit, Japanese persimmon, papaya, guava

Fit it in: Pile on the ketchup and Ragú; guzzle low-sodium V8 and gazpacho; double the amount of tomato paste called for in a recipe.

Pinch hitter: Red and Pink Fruit Bowl: Chop 1 small watermelon, 2 grapefruits, 3 persimmons, 1 papaya, and 4 guavas. Garnish with mint.

CARROTS

What they're great for: fighting cancer, boosting immunity, eyesight

Most red, yellow, or orange vegetables and fruits are spiked with carotenoids, which are fat-soluble compounds that are associated with a reduction in a wide range of cancers, as well as reduced risk and severity of inflammatory conditions such as asthma and rheumatoid arthritis. But none are as easy to prepare, or have as low a caloric density, as carrots.

Aim for: One-half cup a day.

Substitutes: Sweet potato, pumpkin, butternut squash, yellow bell pepper, mango

Fit it in: Raw baby carrots, sliced raw yellow pepper, butternut squash soup, baked sweet potato, pumpkin pie, mango sorbet, carrot cake

Pinch hitter: Baked Sweet Potato Fries: Scrub and dry 2 sweet potatoes. Cut each into eight slices, and then toss with olive oil and paprika. Spread on a baking sheet and bake for 15 minutes at 350°F. Turn and bake for 10 minutes more.

BLUEBERRIES

What they're great for: brainpower, fighting cancer, heart health, boosting immunity

Host to more antioxidants than any other popular fruit, blueberries help prevent cancer, diabetes, and age-related memory changes (hence the nickname "brain berry"). Studies show that blueberries, which are rich in fiber and vitamins A and C, boost cardiovascular health.

Aim for: 1 cup of fresh blueberries a day, or $\frac{1}{2}$ cup frozen or dried.

Substitutes: Açai berries, purple grapes, prunes, raisins, strawberries

Fit it in: Blueberries maintain most of their power in dried, frozen, or jam form.

Pinch hitter: Açai, an Amazonian berry, has even more antioxidants than the blueberry. Mix 2 tablespoons of açai powder into orange juice or add 2 tablespoons of açai pulp to cereal, yogurt, or a smoothie.

BLACK BEANS

What they're great for: muscle growth, brainpower, heart health

All beans are good for your heart, but none can boost your brainpower like black beans. That's because they're full of anthocyanins, which are antioxidant compounds that have been shown to improve brain function.

Aim for: A daily $\frac{1}{2}$-cup serving, which provides 8 grams of protein and 7.5 grams of fiber and is low in calories and free of saturated fat.

Substitutes: Peas, lentils, and pinto, kidney, fava, and lima beans

Fit it in: Wrap black beans in a breakfast burrito; use both black beans and kidney beans in your chili; puree 1 cup of black beans with $\frac{1}{4}$ cup of olive oil and roasted garlic for a healthy dip; add favas, limas, or peas to pasta dishes.

Home run: Black Bean and Tomato Salsa: Dice 4 tomatoes, 1 onion, 3 cloves of garlic, 2 jalapeño peppers, 1 yellow bell pepper, and 1 mango. Mix in a can of black beans and garnish with $\frac{1}{2}$ cup of chopped cilantro and the juice of 2 limes.

WALNUTS

What they're great for: muscle growth, brainpower, fighting cancer, heart health, boosting immunity

Richer in heart-healthy omega-3s than salmon, loaded with more anti-inflammatory polyphenols than red wine, and packing half as much muscle-building protein as chicken, the walnut sounds like a Frankenfood, but it grows on trees. Other nuts combine only one or two of these features, not all three.

Aim for: A serving of walnuts—about 1 ounce, or seven nuts—is good anytime, but especially as a postworkout recovery snack.

Substitutes: Almonds, peanuts, pistachios, macadamia nuts, hazelnuts

Fit it in: Sprinkle on top of salads; dice and add to pancake batter; spoon peanut butter into curries; grind and mix with olive oil to make a marinade for grilled fish or chicken.

Home run: Mix 1 cup of walnuts with $\frac{1}{2}$ cup of dried blueberries and $\frac{1}{4}$ cup of dark chocolate chunks.

OATS

What they're great for: muscle growth, brainpower, heart health

The éminence grise of health food, oats garnered the FDA's first seal of approval. They are packed with soluble fiber, which lowers the risk of heart disease.

Aim for: Yes, oats are loaded with carbs, but the release of those sugars is slowed by the fiber, and because oats also have 10 grams of protein per $\frac{1}{2}$-cup serving, they deliver steady muscle-building energy.

Substitutes: Quinoa, flaxseed, wild rice

Fit it in: Eat granolas and cereals that have a fiber content of at least 5 grams per serving. Sprinkle 2 tablespoons of ground flaxseed on cereals, salads, and yogurt.

Pinch hitter: Quinoa Salad: Quinoa has twice the protein of most cereals and fewer carbs. Boil 1 cup of quinoa in a mixture of 1 cup of pear juice and 1 cup of water. Let cool. In a large bowl, toss 2 diced apples, 1 cup of fresh blueberries, $\frac{1}{2}$ cup of chopped walnuts, and 1 cup of plain fat-free yogurt.

All-Star Panel: Joy Bauer, author of *Joy Bauer's Food Cures* and nutrition advisor on NBC's *Today* show; Laurie Erickson, award-winning wellness chef at Georgia's Sea Island resort; David Heber, MD, PhD, author of *What Color Is Your Diet?*; and Steven Pratt, MD, author of the best-selling *SuperFoods Rx*

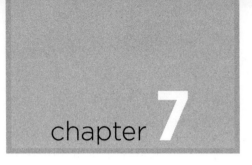

chapter **7**

THE 10 BEST FOODS YOU AREN'T EATING

Do your body a world of good
by expanding your grocery list

Although some people aren't opposed to smoking some weed, most wouldn't think of eating one. It's a shame, really, because a succulent weed named purslane is not only delicious but is also among the world's healthiest foods.

Of course, there are many superfoods that never see the inside of a shopping cart. Some you've never heard of, and others you've simply forgotten about. That's why we've rounded up the best of the bunch. Make a place for them on your table, and you'll instantly upgrade your health—without a prescription.

GOJI BERRIES

These raisin-size fruits are chewy and taste like a cross between a cranberry and a cherry. More important, these potent berries have been used as a medicinal food in Tibet for more than 1,700 years.

Why they're healthy: Goji berries have one of the highest ORAC ratings—a method of gauging antioxidant power—of any fruit, according to Tufts University researchers. And although modern scientists began to study this ancient berry only recently, they've found that the sugars that make goji berries sweet reduce insulin resistance—a risk factor of diabetes—in rats.

How to eat them: Mix dried or fresh goji berries with a cup of plain yogurt, sprinkle them onto your oatmeal or cold cereal, or enjoy a handful by themselves. You can find them at specialty supermarkets or at www.gojiberries.us.

CINNAMON

This old-world spice usually reaches most people's stomachs only when it's mixed with sugar and stuck to a roll.

Why it's healthy: Cinnamon helps control your blood sugar, which influences your risk of heart disease. In fact, USDA researchers found that people with type 2 diabetes who consumed 1 gram of cinnamon a day for 6 weeks (about $\frac{1}{4}$ teaspoon each day) significantly reduced not only their blood sugar but also their triglycerides and low-density lipoproteins (LDL—bad) cholesterol. Credit the spice's active ingredients, methylhydroxychalcone polymers, which increase your cells' ability to metabolize sugar by up to 20 times.

How to eat it: You don't need the fancy oils and extracts sold at vitamin stores; just sprinkle the stuff that's in your spice rack (or in the shaker at Starbucks) into your coffee or onto your oatmeal.

BEETS

These grungy-looking roots are naturally sweeter than any other vegetable, which means they pack tons of flavor underneath their rugged exterior.

Why they're healthy: Think of beets as red spinach. Just like Popeye's powerfood, this crimson vegetable is one of the best sources of both folate and betaine. These two nutrients work together to lower your blood levels of homocysteine, which is an inflammatory compound that can damage your arteries and increase your risk of heart disease. Plus, the natural pigments—called betacyanins—that give beets their color have been proved to be potent cancer fighters in laboratory mice.

How to eat them: Enjoy them fresh and raw, not from a jar. Heating beets actually decreases their antioxidant power. For a simple single-serving salad, wash and peel one beet, and then grate it on the widest blade of a box grater. Toss with 1 tablespoon of olive oil and the juice of half a lemon.

You can eat the leaves and stems, which are also packed with vitamins, minerals, and antioxidants. Simply cut off the stems just below the point where the leaves start, and wash thoroughly. They're now ready to be used in a salad. Or, for a side dish, sauté the leaves, along with a minced clove of garlic and a tablespoon of olive oil, in a pan over medium-high heat. Cook until the leaves are wilted and the stems are tender. Season with salt and pepper and a squeeze of lemon juice, and sprinkle with fresh Parmesan cheese.

CABBAGE

Absent from most American kitchens, this cruciferous vegetable is a major player in European and Asian diets.

Why it's healthy: One cup of chopped cabbage has just 22 calories, and it's loaded with valuable nutrients. At the top of the list is sulforaphane, which is a chemical that increases your body's production of enzymes that disarm cell-damaging free radicals and reduce your risk of cancer. In fact, Stanford University scientists determined that sulforaphane boosts your levels of these cancer-fighting enzymes higher than any other plant chemical.

How to eat it: Put cabbage on your burgers to add a satisfying crunch. Or, for an even better sandwich topping or side salad, try an Asian-style slaw. Here's what you'll need:

4 tablespoons peanut or canola oil

Juice of 2 limes

1 tablespoon sriracha, an Asian chili sauce you can find in the international section of your grocery store

1 head napa cabbage, finely chopped or shredded

$\frac{1}{4}$ cup toasted peanuts

$\frac{1}{2}$ cup shredded carrots

$\frac{1}{4}$ cup chopped cilantro

Whisk together the oil, lime juice, and sriracha. Combine the remaining ingredients in a large mixing bowl and toss with the dressing to coat. Refrigerate for 20 minutes before serving. The slaw will keep in your fridge for 2 days.

GUAVA

Guava is an obscure tropical fruit that's subtly acidic, with sweetness that intensifies as you eat your way to the center.

Why it's healthy: Guava has a higher concentration of lycopene, which is an anti-oxidant that fights prostate cancer, than any other plant food, including tomatoes and watermelon. In addition, 1 cup of the stuff provides 688 milligrams of potassium, which is 63 percent more than you'll find in a medium-size banana. And guava may be the ultimate high-fiber food: There's almost 9 grams of fiber in every cup.

How to eat it: Down the entire fruit, from the rind to the seeds. It's all edible—and nutritious. The rind alone has more vitamin C than you'd find in the flesh of an orange. You can purchase guava in the produce section of higher-end supermarkets or in Latin grocery stores.

SWISS CHARD

Hidden in the leafy-greens cooler of your market, you'll find this slightly bitter, salty vegetable, which is actually native to the Mediterranean.

Why it's healthy: A half cup of cooked Swiss chard provides a huge amount of both lutein and zeaxanthin, supplying 10 milligrams each. These plant chemicals, known as carotenoids, protect your retinas from the damage of aging, according to Harvard researchers. That's because both nutrients, which are actually pigments, appear to accumulate in your retinas, where they absorb the type of shortwave light rays that can damage your eyes. So the more lutein and zeaxanthin you eat, the better your internal eye protection will be.

How to eat it: Chard goes great with grilled steaks and chicken, and it also works well

Antioxidants, Explained

The science is clear: Plant foods are good for you. And the credit often goes to chemicals they produce called *antioxidants*. Just as the name suggests, antioxidants help protect your cells against oxidation. Think of oxidation as rust. This rust is caused by free radicals, which are unstable oxygen atoms that attack your cells, inducing DNA damage that leads to cancer. Thankfully, antioxidants help stabilize free radicals, which keeps the rogue atoms from harming your cells.

So by eating more antioxidant-rich foods, you'll boost the amount of disease-fighting chemicals floating in your bloodstream. The result: Every bite fortifies your body with all-natural preventive medicine.

---

as a bed for pan-seared fish. Wash and dry a bunch of Swiss chard, and then chop the leaves and stems into 1-inch pieces. Heat a tablespoon of olive oil in a large sauté pan or wok, and add two garlic cloves that you've peeled and lightly crushed. When the oil smokes lightly, add the chard. Sauté for 5 to 7 minutes, until the leaves wilt and the stems are tender. Remove the garlic cloves, and season the chard with salt and pepper.

PURSLANE

Although the FDA classifies purslane as a broad-leaved weed, it's a popular vegetable and herb in many other countries, including China, Mexico, and Greece.

Why it's healthy: Purslane has the highest amount of heart-healthy omega-3 fats of any edible plant, according to researchers at the University of Texas at San Antonio. The scientists also report that this herb has 10 to 20 times more melatonin, which is an antioxidant that may inhibit cancer growth, than any other fruit or vegetable tested.

How to eat it: Purslane is a great alternative or addition to lettuce in a salad: The leaves and stems are crisp, chewy, and succulent, and they have a mild lemony taste. Look for it at your local farmer's market or Chinese or Mexican market. It's also available at some Whole Foods stores, as an individual leafy green or in premade salad mixes.

POMEGRANATE JUICE

A popular drink for decades in the Middle East, pomegranate juice has become widely available only recently in the United States.

Why it's healthy: Israeli scientists discovered that people who downed just 2 ounces of pomegranate juice daily for a year decreased their systolic (top number) blood pressure by 21 percent and significantly improved blood flow to their hearts. What's more, 4 ounces provides 50 percent of your daily vitamin C needs.

How to drink it: Try 100 percent pomegranate juice from Pom Wonderful. It contains no added sugars, and because it's so powerful, a small glassful is all you need. (For a list of retailers, go to www.pomwonderful.com.)

DRIED PLUMS

You may know these better by the moniker "prunes," which are indelibly linked with nursing homes and bathroom habits. And that explains why, in an effort to revive this delicious fruit's image, producers now market them under another name.

Why they're healthy: Prunes contain high amounts of neochlorogenic and chlorogenic acids, antioxidants that are particularly effective at combating the "superoxide anion radical." This nasty free radical causes structural damage to your cells, and such damage is thought to be one of the primary causes of cancer.

How to eat them: As an appetizer. Wrap a paper-thin slice of prosciutto around each dried plum and secure with a toothpick. Bake in a 400°F oven for 10 to 15 minutes, until the plums are soft and the prosciutto is crispy. Most of the fat will cook off, and you'll be left with a decadent-tasting treat that's sweet, savory, and healthy.

PUMPKIN SEEDS

These jack-o'-lantern waste products are the most nutritious part of the pumpkin.

Why they're healthy: Downing pumpkin seeds is the easiest way to consume more magnesium. That's important because French researchers recently determined that people with the highest levels of magnesium in their blood have a 40 percent lower risk of early death than those with the lowest levels. And on average, men in particular consume 353 milligrams of the mineral daily, well under the 420-milligram minimum recommended by the USDA.

How to eat them: Whole, shells and all. (The shells provide extra fiber.) Roasted pumpkin seeds contain 150 milligrams of magnesium per ounce. Add them to your regular diet, and you'll easily hit your daily target of 420 milligrams. Look for them in the snack or health food section of your grocery store, next to the peanuts, almonds, and sunflower seeds.

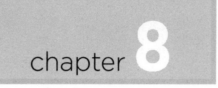

chapter 8

FIVE FOOD RULES TO BREAK

Don't let your diet—or stomach—be held captive by these nutrition myths

It goes like this: A client looking to lead a healthier life hires a nutritionist to help him improve his diet. The nutritionist analyzes what the man has been eating and factors in his food preferences, and together they create an eating plan that fits his lifestyle and goals. Soon after, the client is noticeably leaner and more energetic—a happy customer.

That's when the trouble starts. After a coworker asks the man for the details of his diet, the client suddenly finds himself in a heated interrogation. Doesn't your nutritionist know that red meat causes cancer? And that potatoes cause diabetes? Shouldn't he tell you to eat less salt to prevent high blood pressure?

It's enough to make the man throw up his hands and head to the nearest drive-thru. Nutrition misinformation fools people into being confused and frustrated in their quest to eat healthily, even if they're already achieving great results. Thankfully, you're about to be enlightened by science. Here are five food fallacies that you can forget about for good.

MYTH #1: "HIGH PROTEIN INTAKE IS HARMFUL TO YOUR KIDNEYS"

The origin: Back in 1983, researchers first discovered that eating more protein increases your glomerular filtration rate (GFR). Think of GFR as the amount of blood your kidneys are filtering per minute. From this finding, many scientists made the leap that a higher GFR places your kidneys under greater stress.

The science: Nearly 2 decades ago, Dutch researchers found that although a protein-rich meal did boost GFR, it didn't have an adverse effect on overall kidney function. In fact, there's zero published research showing that downing hefty amounts of protein—specifically, up to 1.27 grams per pound of body weight a day—damages healthy kidneys.

The bottom line: As a rule of thumb, shoot to eat your target body weight in grams of protein daily. For example, if you weigh 200 pounds but want to get down to 180, then eat 180 grams of protein a day.

In Defense of Butter

Sure, butter is rich in fat—especially the saturated kind. But most of this fat is composed of palmitic and stearic acids. Research shows these saturated fatty acids either have no effect on your cholesterol or actually improve it. Not enough to convince you that butter—in moderation, of course—isn't a dietary demon? Keep reading.

One pat of butter contains just 36 calories, and the fat it provides helps you feel full longer.

Butter is one of the top sources of conjugated linoleic acid (CLA), which is a natural fat that's been shown to fight cancer.

Studies show that the fat in butter improves your body's ability to absorb vitamins A, E, D, and K. So a pat of butter on your vegetables actually makes them healthier (and tastier).

MYTH #2: "SWEET POTATOES ARE BETTER FOR YOU THAN WHITE POTATOES ARE"

The origin: Because most Americans eat the highly processed version of the white potato—for instance, french fries and potato chips—consumption of this root vegetable has been linked to obesity and an increased diabetes risk. Meanwhile, sweet potatoes, which are typically eaten whole, have been celebrated for being rich in nutrients and also having a lower glycemic index than their white brethren.

The science: White potatoes and sweet potatoes have complementary nutritional differences; one isn't necessarily better than the other. For instance, sweet potatoes have more fiber and vitamin A, but white potatoes are higher in essential minerals, such as iron, magnesium, and potassium. As for the glycemic index, sweet potatoes are lower on the scale, but baked white potatoes typically aren't eaten without cheese, sour cream, or butter. These toppings all contain fat, which lowers the glycemic index of a meal.

The bottom line: The form in which you consume a potato—for instance, a whole baked potato versus a processed potato that's used to make chips—is more important than the type of spud.

MYTH #3: "RED MEAT CAUSES CANCER"

The origin: In a 1986 study, Japanese researchers discovered cancer developing in rats that were fed heterocyclic amines, compounds that are generated from overcooking meat under high heat. And since then, some studies of large populations have suggested a potential link between meat and cancer.

The science: No study has ever found a direct cause-and-effect relationship between red-meat consumption and cancer. As for the population studies, they're far from conclusive. That's because they rely on broad surveys of people's eating habits and health afflictions, and those numbers are simply crunched to find trends, not causes.

The bottom line: Don't stop grilling. Meat lovers who are worried about the supposed risks of grilled meat don't need to avoid burgers and steak; rather, they should just trim off the burned or overcooked sections of the meat before eating.

MYTH #4: "HIGH-FRUCTOSE CORN SYRUP IS MORE FATTENING THAN REGULAR SUGAR IS"

The origin: In a 1968 study, rats that were fed large amounts of fructose developed high levels of fat in their bloodstreams. Then, in 2002, University of California at Davis researchers published a well-publicized paper noting that Americans' increasing consumption of fructose, including that in high-fructose corn syrup (HFCS), paralleled our skyrocketing rates of obesity.

The science: Both HFCS and sucrose—which is better known as table sugar—contain similar amounts of fructose. For instance, the two most commonly used types of HFCS are HFCS-42 and HFCS-55, which are 42 and 55 percent fructose, respectively. Sucrose is almost chemically identical, containing 50 percent fructose. This is why the University of California at Davis scientists determined fructose intakes from both HFCS and sucrose. The truth is, there's no evidence to show any differences in these two types of sugar. Both will cause weight gain when consumed in excess.

The bottom line: HFCS and regular sugar are empty-calorie carbohydrates that should be consumed in limited amounts. How? By keeping soft drinks, sweetened fruit juices, and prepackaged desserts to a minimum.

MYTH #5: "SALT CAUSES HIGH BLOOD PRESSURE AND SHOULD BE AVOIDED"

The origin: In the 1940s, a Duke University researcher named Walter Kempner, MD, became famous for using salt restriction to treat people with high blood pressure. Later, studies confirmed that reducing salt could help reduce hypertension.

The science: Large-scale scientific reviews have determined there's no reason for people with normal blood pressure to restrict their sodium intake. Now, if you already have high blood pressure, you may be "salt sensitive." As a result, reducing the amount of salt you eat could be helpful.

However, it's been known for the past 20 years that people with high blood pressure who don't want to lower their salt intake can simply consume more potassium-containing foods.

Why? It's really the balance of the two minerals that matters. In fact, Dutch researchers determined that a low potassium intake has the same impact on your blood pressure as high salt consumption does.

The bottom line: Strive for a potassium-rich diet, which you can achieve by eating a wide variety of fruits, vegetables, and legumes. For instance, spinach, broccoli, bananas, white potatoes, and most types of beans each contain more than 400 milligrams of potassium per serving.

chapter 9

HEALTHY FOOD IN A HURRY

New take-out and food delivery services make putting a healthy dinner on the table easy—and affordable

P haedra Hise, a mom in Richmond, Virginia, knew things had gotten out of hand when her 10-year-old begged for a home-cooked meal. "Mommy," she pleaded as Hise was throwing together some ham sandwiches to eat in the car after swim practice, "when are you going to make a real dinner again?"

Hey, it's not like Hise didn't want to. But with work, family, exercise, volunteer obligations, and a dog to walk, she and her husband were always getting home late and starving—a setup for take-out or flung-together sandwiches.

Getting a healthy meal on the table is a major challenge for most people these days. Maybe that's why there has been a boom in new food services—companies that deliver groceries to you, storefronts where you assemble a meal to bring home, and everything in between. Online grocery shopping alone was a $2.4 billion industry in 2004—and is expected to grow to $6.5 billion by 2008.

Anything that promises dinner in record time sounds good to us. But how fast, tasty, and healthy are these services, really? Hise and her family were just the guinea pigs to find out: her daughter, Lily; her 44-year-old husband, Bill; and Hise, an active, harried 42-year-old. For 6 weeks, they explored the world of convenience meals, trying an option each week in their Richmond, Virginia, home. Here's what the meals offered in terms of flavor, nutrition, convenience, and cost.

GROCERIES DELIVERED

The service: You order online—or in some cases via a faxed list—and presto: A couple of days later, your groceries are at your front door. Local markets sometimes offer this option; there are also regional and national companies, including Peapod, NetGrocer, and now Amazon. An important variable: Some deliver anything you can find in your local store, while the national biggies ship only shelf-stable products (no perishables).

How It Worked

When the Hise family lived in Boston a few years ago, they saved a couple of hours a week by using Peapod for grocery deliveries from the nearby Stop & Shop. The service chose fresher produce and meats than the family did and charged just $7 to $10 for next-day delivery. It was lovely to get groceries without dragging a cranky toddler to the store.

Peapod doesn't deliver in their current hometown, so they chose NetGrocer. Unfortunately, this service handles only packaged goods, not fresh food, and it doesn't list label information for some products. That can be a problem, says Cynthia Sass, MPH, RD, *Prevention*'s nutrition director, because canned and boxed foods tend to be high in sodium and fat. (Like NetGrocer, Peapod and Amazon list ingredients for many but not all products.)

Still, Hise was able to do some quick and easy menu planning: pasta and organic jarred tomato sauce (which she would supplement with salad or other fresh vegetables) and soup and grilled cheese sandwiches (ditto).

The delivery fee was an obvious negative, but she put in the plus column the fact that she made fewer impulse buys when shopping online. (With no sample tastings, you can even save on calories.) Probably because Hise was shopping from her desk instead of in a crowded store with a chattering child, she suddenly remembered a simple recipe for a corn tortilla and black bean casserole she hadn't made in years. How convenient, she thought—until the delivery arrived without the beans ("temporarily out of stock"). That reminded her: Peapod asks you when you place your order if substitutions are okay.

MEAL PREP PLACES

The service: When Hise heard about My Girlfriend's Kitchen (MGFK), the very name gave her multilevel marketing jitters. She envisioned being dragged to a meal-assembly "party" and forced to sign up for a year's worth of prepackaged food. Wrong. MGFK (which is now called Dinner A'Fare) and similar companies, such as Let's Do Dinner and Let's Dish!, consist of storefronts where you assemble prechopped and premixed ingredients in the pans or bags they provide. Then you take your stack of ready-to-cook meals home to store in the freezer. This trend is taking off like crazy: Nearly 1,100 meal-assembly kitchens have popped up in the United States and Canada in recent years.

How It Worked

On the MGFK Web site, Hise found a nutritionally detailed list of 14 meals and selected 6. A few days later, she took her daughter to the shop, where they found a dozen different food stations, each stocked with bins of ingredients—mostly frozen but appetizing, with brightly colored veggies, good-looking chicken and fish, and lean, red beef. They went from station to station, following posted instructions to scoop precise amounts into a foil pan or plastic bag: a scoop of ground turkey plus smaller scoops of grated carrots, celery, walnuts, and herbs for Little Meatloaf on the Prairie, for instance. It was fast, taking just over an hour, and easy (really easy, because Hise's daughter ended up elbowing her aside).

They arrived home with instructions on each package and a handy reference list detailing how to cook each meal they loaded into the freezer.

You have to check that list each morning—as Hise discovered a few days later, when she realized just before dinner that I hadn't defrosted Inga's Traditional Swedish Meatballs. That dish required sautéing, but plenty go from the freezer straight into the slow cooker or oven. You also have to cook the pasta or rice that comes with many of the meals, and supplement the entrées with side dishes or salad, if you're so inclined. The food is family friendly (read: accommodating to picky pint-size eaters) and good—better than you get at many casual restaurants, especially because you can add or subtract ingredients according to your taste. Exotic it's not, but Hise has been back three times.

"I call it halfway homemade," says Sass. "The food is pretty much guaranteed to be tasty, but you don't have to go buy a cookbook. On the flip side, some of the dishes can be high in fat and calories."

Detailed nutritional info on many of these services' Web sites can help you avoid those pitfalls. Elisa Zied, RD, an American Diabetes Association (ADA) spokesperson, also recommends boosting the vegetable content of many of the one-dish meals. "Eyeball the vegetable serving," she suggests. "If it's under half a cup, add to it with bagged baby carrots or low-sodium canned vegetables." Because people get most of their veggies at dinner, she says, "it's a good idea to get at least a cup per person."

DINNER FROM AISLE SIX

The service: The salad bar and ready-to-eat sections in supermarkets are growing like weeds: Profits grew 10 percent each year between 2000 and 2005, industry analysts say. And the offerings are getting ever more elaborate—not just salad makings but soup, pizza, hot panini, and sushi—sometimes made to order. And, of course, the ubiquitous roasted chicken.

How It Worked

On a busy night when her husband was out of town, Hise took her daughter, Lily, to their local market. Hise told Lily she could get whatever she wanted, as long as it was loosely based on the food pyramid. She chose three hard-boiled eggs, a cup of green peas, several chunks of watermelon, and a roll (not a traditional mix, but hey, she ate it all). Hise took small portions of various exotic salads, such as Asian chicken, quinoa, and black bean and corn.

Salad bar items are sold by weight, so the dense eggs and heavy watermelon Lily chose really added up; in fact, the meal was slightly more expensive than the one they got later in the week from the sushi bar. Another night, their budget dinner included roasted chicken and raw broccoli, which Hise cooked at home along with rice to round out the meal.

Cost and Convenience

To see how the new options measured up, Hise tracked the time and money she spent cooking meals at home for a week; later, she did the same for takeout. Then we ran the numbers.

OPTION	COST PER SERVING	TIME	OUR RD COMMENTS	FOR MORE INFO
Home Cooking	$3	Time required: 12½ hours (2 in the market and 1½ per day in the kitchen)	Zied gave the meals a thumbs-up. But then, who wouldn't cook nutritious meals with an RD checking the menu?	Call Mom.
Salad Bar	$2.50 to $8	Time saved: About 10¼ hours per week	"Salad bars can be more expensive," Sass says, "but if you choose wisely, you can get five servings of produce in a single meal."	www.whole foods.com (store locator) www.wildoats.com (store locator) your local market
Grocery Delivery	$3.50	Time saved: 2 hours per week if the service includes perishables; otherwise, none	"Love these services, so long as they deliver fresh food. There's less stress and temptation, and you can really shop smart," says Sass.	www.peapod.com www.netgrocer.com www.amazon.com Regionally available: www.freshdirect.com www.safeway.com www.simondelivers.com
Meal Assembly	$4	Time saved: 6½ hours per week	"This is just as good as homemade, without all the work," says Sass. But watch the fat and calories, and supplement with bagged carrots, salad greens, or microwaved frozen veggies.	www.dinnerafare.com www.letsdodinner.biz www.dinnerbydesignkitchen.com www.supersuppers.com
Diet Delivery	$6 to $8	Time saved: About 12 hours per week	"There are better ways to lose weight," says Zied.	www.ediets.com www.chefsdiet.com www.Bistro MD.com www.atkinsathome.com
Local Chef	$6 to $8	Time saved: About 12 hours per week	"These can be good or awful, depending on the chef," says Zied. "Make sure you check out the nutritional info, and talk with the chef, if necessary."	www.personalcheftogo.com www.dinewise.com
Takeout	$9	Time saved: 9 hours	"Too much fat, too many calories, too much sodium, and it makes you feel . . . yuck," Zied says.	www.yellowpages.com

Pricey or not, a salad bar can be a fast way to a healthy dinner. "You can usually find all kinds and colors of veggies, which means more nutrients and phytochemicals," Sass says. "Buying 10 different vegetables to make a salad at home would get pretty expensive, and they'd probably go bad before you used them up."

But keep an eye on the sodium—and calories, warns Zied. A salad bar's crunchy croutons, creamy dressings, and mayo-drenched mélanges are obvious disasters, but you don't want to go overboard even on healthy options such as chickpeas or raisins; stick to about ½ cup of the beans and no more than 2 tablespoons of dried fruit.

What's more, if you're trying to lose weight, it's a good idea to pick just one or two salads, Zied adds; save other tantalizing choices for your next visit. "Research shows that you eat less when there aren't too many tastes competing with each other," she says.

CHEF ON CALL

The service: This "someone-else-cooks-it" category is stocked with gifted (and not so gifted) amateurs and professionals who have tired of interminable restaurant hours. These aren't personal chef services; dishes aren't made to order. Instead, the companies offer daily or weekly menus of fresh-cooked meals delivered to your home, where you pile them into the fridge or freezer.

How It Worked

Hise's local service, Personal Chef To Go, allowed no substitutions, but they didn't mind. They got family-style containers of Zesty Whole Wheat Pasta Bake, Shrimp Scampi over Six-Grain Rice Pilaf, and Oven-Roasted Sliced Lean Filet of Beef, among other entrées—and all of it tasted gourmet. Bonus: There were lots of interesting ingredients, such as roasted red peppers, pesto, and orzo.

Zied was ready to place an order herself. But because companies like this vary widely, she recommends looking for one that posts nutrient analyses. "Otherwise, who knows how much butter the chef is throwing in?" she asks.

And even when the info is on the Web site, look for what isn't there—such as sodium (it wasn't listed on Hise's nutritional information). "Just call up and talk with the chef," she advises.

DIET FOOD BY MAIL

The service: Plenty of online companies ship fresh meals, most of them to people who want to lose weight. Typically, these outfits aren't simply dinner providers; they send you food for the whole day. Some give you a choice of entrées, but generally a weekly prix fixe menu is much less pricey.

How It Worked

Hise's idea of heaven is to pop a plate of something nutritious and delicious into the microwave oven and sit down to dinner 3 minutes later. So she was charmed when she heard about eDiets Express, which promised to let her choose a week's worth of breakfasts, lunches, dinners, and snacks for delivery. But when she ordered, a message popped up: The first week of meals was preselected, no changes allowed. She received stuffed peppers with a side of vegetables, boneless baked chicken with beets, and turkey meat loaf with chickpea salad, among other dishes. She also got muffins. A lot of muffins. In fact, that was all she got for breakfast 2 out of the 7 days they used the service.

Zied was not impressed. "What's with the muffins? A blueberry muffin is not a meal. Breakfast is your best opportunity to get four key elements: whole grains, fiber, dairy, and fruit. This skimps on all of them, and the rest of the day looks just as bad."

Hise loved the convenience, but that was about all eDiets had going for it. The stuffed peppers tasted okay, but the chicken breast was flavorless and rubbery, and they had to douse the turkey meat loaf in ketchup. Plus, the portions were too small.

The meal plan will work for weight loss and maintenance, according to eDiets, but the maximum calories offered are a mere 1,400 per day. That's not enough for a 220-pound man; even a reasonably active woman of Hise's height (5-foot-6) should be getting about 1,800 calories, Zied says. By the second day, they all were starving. The eDiets dietitian told Hise that they should each add 800 to 1,000 calories per day in snacks—which they had to provide.

"This isn't really helpful for a dieter," Zied says. "You could pick junk food for those 800 calories. You wouldn't get the nutrients you need, and you'd probably still end up hungry. Basically, you have to become your own dietitian."

Exchange Changes ————————————————————

If you have diabetes, you're likely very familiar with the diabetes exchanges. The exchange lists were established by a joint project with the American Diabetes Association, the American Dietetic Association, and US Public Health Service in 1950, explained the American Diabetes Association's president-elect, health care and education, Sue McLaughlin, BS, RD, CDE, CPT.

In 2008, the ADA updated their exchange lists as follows:

- Eliminated the Very Lean Meat group by folding it into the existing Lean Meat group.
- Established the plant protein group Meat Substitutes.
- Added a category in the Milk group for dairylike foods, such as soy and rice milk.
- Pulled fat-free salad dressings into the Other Carbs list or into the Free Foods, but labeled them as modified fat foods with carbohydrate.

Also, the ADA has recently developed a free online tool, MyFoodAdvisor, that is based on the exchange lists, McLaughlin said. The serving sizes for foods in the database are based on consistent amounts of carbohydrate, protein and fat to help individuals with diabetes, or those without who want to make healthful food choices, easily compare foods. MyFoodAdvisor allows you to compare two foods, request healthier options, and use the "create a dish" to tally all that you eat in a day for a grand total of calories, fat, carbohydrate, sodium, and 16 other nutrients.

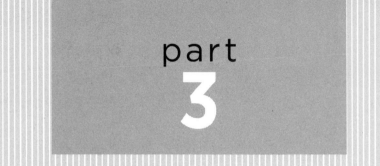

part
3

LOSE WEIGHT

medical BREAKTHROUGHS

Here's the latest research on the weight loss front.

GET SOME MOTIVATION

More than two-thirds of Americans are overweight or obese. More than 8 percent of us have diabetes. A connection? Absolutely.

To add more links to this connection, researchers at the University of Missouri studied 21 women and 9 men who were overweight or obese but whose weight was stable. At the beginning of the study, the scientists gave all participants a physical and drew their blood. For the next 6 months, the volunteers followed a strict meal plan and exercise regimen. At the end of the study, the scientists drew more blood.

The researchers discovered that the volunteers who had lost 10 percent or more of their weight showed significant improvements in their ability to handle insulin. Weight loss can help the body handle insulin, the scientists concluded.

According to the American Diabetes Association (ADA), reducing your body weight by even 5 to 7 percent (which is generally about 10 to 15 pounds) and exercising for 2½ hours each week can help reduce your risk of developing diabetes by 58 percent.

TALK IT OUT

Think one counseling session can't make a difference? Think again. Researchers in Switzerland randomly chose almost 4,000 overweight people who had been screened in pharmacies for diabetes. The researchers divided the people into three groups. The first group received standard counseling, without specific recommendations to make lifestyle changes. The second group received counseling plus advice to reduce their weight. The third group received counseling, advice to reduce their weight, and the recommendation to contact a physician.

Three months later, all the people had lost significant amounts of weight, and the two groups that received advice to reduce the weight lost the most. The scientists concluded that counseling in community pharmacies after screening for diabetes can result in significant lifestyle changes and weight loss in people who are overweight.

PARE DOWN

Apple body types are becoming less and less "apeeling." Past studies have shown that people with apple-shaped physiques are at greater risk for diabetes, clogged arteries, and high blood pressure .

More recently, researchers at the National Institutes of Health and Harvard Medical School studied more than 44,000 women for 16 years. The scientists discovered that middle-aged or older women who carried their weight in their middles, with a waistline of 35 inches or more—were more than twice as likely to die of heart disease and had a 63 percent higher risk of cancer than women with waistlines less than 28 inches. This was regardless of their weight; even normal-weight women with waistlines greater than 35 inches had a greater risk of dying from heart disease or stroke.

These results are particularly sobering for people with diabetes because more than 65 percent of people with diabetes die from heart disease or stroke, according to the ADA.

CUT DOWN POUNDS

Japanese researchers recently proved what dietitians have been saying for years: Slicing your food into strips or chunks may help you eat less. Study participants who compared equal amounts of sliced and whole vegetables rated the sliced serving as much as 27 percent larger.

The end result: Believing that you are eating a larger portion of food causes you to feel more satisfied with fewer calories, according to Kaoru Kohyama, PhD, the study author. Stack your slices. The taller the food sits on your plate, the more appetizing it will seem.

BE A SLOB

Keeping your dirty dishes or empty glasses in view can help you control overeating. When researchers at Cornell University treated graduate students to a free chicken-wing buffet, those whose dishes piled up ate 28 percent less than people whose tables were continually bused. The people who ate more thought they were hungrier because they didn't have a visual cue to keep their appetite in check.

"Whether you're eating chicken wings or cookies, you'll have less if you see evidence of what you've already eaten," says Brian Wansink, PhD, director of Cornell's Food and Brand Lab and author of *Mindless Eating*.

DRINK FEWER CALORIES

We have a national drinking problem: Americans consume 21 percent of their daily calories from beverages, according to researchers from the University of North Carolina at Chapel Hill. Lighten up without losing the flavor of your favorite cool thirst quenchers.

Instead of a 17.5-ounce strawberry smoothie (290 calories), go for a 16-ounce Jamba Juice Jamba Light Strawberry Nirvana smoothie with real fruit (150 calories) for a daily savings of 140 calories, which is enough to lose 15 pounds in 1 year.

Instead of a 16-ounce lemonade (220 calories), go for a 15.2-ounce Tropicana Fruit Squeeze Summer Lemon (35 calories) for a daily savings of 185 calories, which is enough to lower your body mass index (BMI) by an average of 2 points in 6 months.

Instead of a 12-ounce chai iced tea latte (200 calories), go for a 8-ounce iced brewed chai tea with 2 tablespoons of fat-free milk (11 calories), for a daily savings of 189 calories, which is equal to eating 1 less slice of pizza.

Instead of a 16-ounce peach iced tea (200 calories), go for a 16-ounce Inko's White Unsweetened Honeysuckle iced tea (0 calories), for a daily savings of 200 calories, which is the amount you'd save by not eating 1 chocolate-frosted doughnut.

Instead of a 16-ounce orange soda (238 calories), go for a 16-ounce Nestlé Pure Life Tropical Fruit Splash flavored water (0 calories), for a daily savings of 238 calories, which is the amount you'd burn in 60 minutes of 3-mph pace walking.

Note, all calculations are based on a 150-pound person. If you weigh less, you'll burn fewer calories; if you weigh more, you'll burn more calories.

CHEW ON THIS

A new kind of gum may really help drop pounds. Researchers at the Imperial College London are developing a gum using a drug based on the satiety-signaling hormone pancreatic polypeptide. They injected either the hormone or a placebo into 10 overweight people and offered them a buffet. The people who received the hormone ate 22 percent less at lunch and 25 percent fewer calories over the next 24 hours. The gum should be available in 5 to 10 years.

HEAT IT UP

Capsaicin, the compound that heats up a chile pepper, may also help keep off pounds, according to a study in the *Journal of Agricultural and Food Chemistry*. When scientists exposed fat cells to capsaicin in a lab, the cells died. It's hard to say if the spice has the same effect in humans, but we can hope! If tongue-tingling condiments overwhelm your palate, try Dave's Gourmet Adjustable Heat Hot Sauce ($10; www.davesgourmet.com)—a twist of the cap turns a serving of sauce from slightly spicy to downright fiery (or somewhere in between).

DIAL AWAY POUNDS

To lose extra pudge, plan phone dates with a dietitian. A new study shows that almost 80 percent of people say professional phone therapy gave them better results from diet and exercise. Try one of the following plans that incorporate phone counseling.

Program: Jenny Craig

Cost: $20–$199 for 6 months

Phone time included: 15–20 minutes each week

Program: eDiets.com

Cost: $18 per month

Phone time included: Unlimited

Program: NutriSystem

Cost: $294–$326

Phone time included: Unlimited

LOSE 7 POUNDS WITHOUT TRYING

You don't have to work out longer to burn more calories and get the fit body you want. Fold these tricks into your routine five times a week to drop 3 to 7 pounds in a year without logging an extra minute of exercise.

Bonus burn: 50 calories

Walk with poles to zap 20 percent more calories and tone your upper body.

Push yourself to pedal just 2 mph faster during half of a cycling workout.

Bonus burn: 75 calories

Add 10 1-minute bouts of jogging to your walk.

Alternate upper and lower body rather than resting between moves, and do two sets instead of one.

Bonus burn: 100 calories

Turn your weight workout into a circuit by doing jumping jacks rather than resting between exercises.

Spend half your treadmill workout on a 5 percent incline.

Note, all calculations are based on a 150-pound person. If you weigh less, you'll burn fewer calories; if you weigh more, you'll burn more calories.

CHECK YOUR OIL

Start your exercise session with a shot of oil. Regular exercise combined with fish-oil supplements results in fat loss, reports the *American Journal of Clinical Nutrition*. Researchers had 65 overweight people take 6 grams daily of either fish oil or sunflower oil. Half the people in each group ran or walked three times a week for 45 minutes. After 12 weeks, the fish-oil eaters who exercised had lost 3.3 pounds on average; the others saw only minor weight loss.

Both exercise and fish oil increase the activity of fat-burning enzymes, so combining them leads to greater fat loss, says researcher Alison Hill, PhD. To boost your burn: Pop 2 grams of flavored fish-oil capsules 2 hours before your workout.

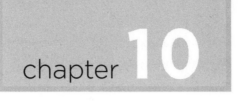

chapter **10**

WEIGHT LOSS FOR HEALTHY EATERS

Try these subtle diet tweaks for real results

You snack on fruit, check calorie counts, and start most days with a walk or swim. So when you step on that scale and the needle stays put, you wonder what the heck you're doing wrong. Even with such healthy habits, sometimes a seemingly inconsequential snack choice or a larger (but common) food myth can keep pounds in place. Take heart: A simple, slight adjustment in how you eat and think can help you reach your weight loss goal.

HEALTHY HABIT: YOU COUNT CALORIES

Take in fewer calories than your body needs to maintain your current weight, and you will drop pounds. But only 11 percent of Americans correctly estimate their ideal daily calorie requirements, according to a recent survey. The rest of us tend to overestimate, says Bonnie Taub-Dix, RD, a spokesperson for the American Dietetic Association, and that's what keeps you from losing weight. Let's say you assume that a target of 2,000 calories per day will allow you to get to your weight goal, but it really takes 1,800: Those extra 200 are enough to keep an additional 20 pounds on your frame.

Do it better: Determine the right number of calories you need each day—and stick to it. Go to www.prevention.com/caloriecalculator and plug in the weight you want to be (as well as your height, age, and activity level) to get your daily calorie allowance. Set limits on your meals and snacks. If 1,800 calories is your max, split it into three 500-calorie meals and one 300-calorie snack. Create a custom meal. If your favorite frozen entrée has 500 calories, that's all you get. Find one for 300, however, and you can have some fresh fruit and a small salad with it.

HEALTHY HABIT: YOU'RE CONSISTENTLY ACTIVE

Spend a few hours running errands, and it feels like you've worked off some serious weight. But even between-the-aisle laps at the mall, hauling around shopping bags, and loading and unloading the car, you burned only about 400 calories—that's about $\frac{1}{10}$ of a pound.

Do it better: Rev your routine. Short bursts of intense activity burn more calories—and up to 36 percent more fat, according to a recent study published in the *Journal of Applied Physiology*. Strolling around the mall or the park for an hour works off about 150 calories; pick up the pace 1 minute out of every 5 to burn over one-third more calories (try a similar method if you bike). Swimmers can switch from freestyle or breaststroke to a more challenging crawl every few laps, or just go a little faster. Even small steps make a difference: Skip the elevator and carry your groceries up the stairs to burn 128 more calories, or instead of hitting an automatic car wash, do it yourself and zap 204 calories.

HEALTHY HABIT: YOU CHOOSE NUTRITIOUS FOODS

What you put on your plate is important, but healthy eating is also about being mindful of how much you consume. For example, your husband has pancakes with butter and syrup for breakfast, your son grabs a doughnut, and you opt for a cup of oatmeal with a handful of walnuts, a sliced banana, and a large glass of organic blueberry juice. You may win on nutrients, but when it comes to calories you're dead last: That healthy-

At the Restaurant: Five "Healthy" Foods to Avoid

Wheat pancakes: Ounce for ounce, pancakes made with buckwheat and whole wheat flour have the same number of calories as the plain old buttermilk type. Save calories by skipping the butter and syrup.

Taco salad: Eat the edible shell and you'll consume nearly twice as many calories than if you eat the salad alone. Reduce temptation. Order yours on a regular plate.

Soup in a bread bowl: The same theory applies to soup: The edible bowl adds more than 550 calories to your total count. Opting for oyster crackers is a little better, but ½ cup is still 96 additional calories.

Vegetable quesadilla: It has about the same number of calories as the chicken version; the reason is often the cheese, so ask the server to hold half.

Fish sandwich: Even without the tartar sauce, a breaded fish patty at a fast-food restaurant has more calories than a bacon cheeseburger. Go for whatever is grilled.

---

sounding meal adds up to almost 700, more than a third of your allotment for the day.

Do it better: Keep portions of even healthy foods in check. The best way to know if you're eating too much is to write it down. "Even if you note it on a napkin and then throw it away, that's okay. Just the act of writing makes you more aware," says Taub-Dix. Portion control cues help, too: a baseball-size serving for chopped veggies and fruits; a golf ball for nuts and shredded cheese; a fist for rice and pasta; and a deck of cards for lean meats. Also, swap higher-calorie healthy foods for high-fiber, lower-cal varieties like the following:

Fruit: A ½-cup serving of strawberries has 23 calories, while a medium banana has more than 100. An orange has almost half the calories of a glass of orange juice. More low-cal picks include melon and blueberries.

Vegetables: Per 1 cup, raw spinach has 7 calories and boiled eggplant contains 35 calories; mashed sweet potato, however, has 249.

Whole grains: Two full cups of air-popped popcorn (a whole grain) has about the same number of calories as three little whole wheat crackers.

HEALTHY HABIT: YOU ORDER THE HEALTHIEST-SOUNDING ITEM ON THE MENU

Choose the turkey sandwich over pizza and you think you're being good, but again, looks can be deceiving. A turkey sandwich at Panera Bread comes on focaccia with cheese and mayo and delivers 960 calories. Two slices of pepperoni pan pizza from Pizza Hut total 560 calories. Put your sandwich in a spinach wrap instead of regular bread? It's the same difference, says Tara Gidus, RD, a spokesperson for the American Diabetes Association. "My clients think they get more nutrients and save on calories with 'healthy bread,' but often that's not the case."

Do it better: Look up fast-food nutrition facts in advance. Many restaurants offer nutrition information, from Taco Bell to Subway. See if your favorite eatery has nutrition facts online or in the store. You may be surprised at what you see. We were when we checked out Baskin Robbins: A medium strawberry-banana smoothie has 80 more calories than a strawberry milk shake! (See "Five 'Healthy' Foods to Avoid" on page 91 for more diet surprises.)

HEALTHY HABIT: YOU SATISFY CRAVINGS WITH "DIET" TREATS

When you want something sweet, all those fat-free, sugar-free options seem like a smart idea. But researchers at Cornell University found that overweight people who choose low-fat versions of snack foods rather than the regular kinds consume on average twice as many calories.

"The terms *fat-free* and *sugar-free* can create a green light effect, triggering people to eat more," says Cynthia Sass, MPH, RD, *Prevention*'s nutrition director. But many fat-free foods have about the same number of calories (or more) as their full-fat counterparts. Case in point: One variety of oatmeal-raisin cookie has 107 calories and 9 grams of sugar, and the fat-free version of the same brand has 106 calories and 14 grams of sugar.

Do it better: Go for reasonable amounts of the real thing. If you adore ice cream, have a small scoop of premium. "You won't stick to a diet that doesn't include your favorites," says David Grotto, RD, a spokesperson for the American Dietetic Association. Bottom line: Life's too short for forbidden foods.

chapter 11

WEEKEND DIET WISDOM

Stick with it—Monday through Sunday—
to lose weight and keep it off

There's something about weekends that sends caution—and calories—to the wind. Even if your workweek is all about smart snacks and sensible dinners, for many of us, all bets are off come 5 p.m. Friday, says clinical psychologist Robert Maurer, PhD, author of *One Small Step Can Change Your Life*. "It's almost like a dam bursting," he says. We're tired and feel like we've earned the right to put healthy habits on hold. A University of North Carolina at Chapel Hill study revealed that adults take in an extra 222 calories over the course of the weekend (including Friday).

Of course, you want to live a little on the weekend, but if you're trying to lose weight, or even just keep the scale steady, you have to maintain a certain level of vigilance. Here's how to rethink your weekend habits so you'll lose weight all week.

Weekend think: This week was tough; I deserve to splurge.

Healthier splurge: Splurge with extra savvy.

The need for a reward is human nature, says Stephen Gullo, PhD, author of *The Thin*

Commandments Diet. And for many, that "something special" is food. You can't change what makes you happy, but you can minimize the diet damage. Choose one portion-controlled item that requires you to leave the house, such as a cup of lobster bisque from your favorite eatery or a small, fresh pastry from the bakery. "It's more rewarding to have a nice treat than to waste calories on regular things you can have anytime, like potato chips or cookies," says Gullo. Doing something special works, too: Catch a movie or get a massage.

Weekend think: Eating and entertaining go hand in hand.

Healthier splurge: Plan some activities, not meals.

When you eat with friends, you consume 50 percent more than you do alone, found a Pennsylvania State University study. Researchers suspect that it's not the food but a tendency to lengthen the meal to keep the good times going. Instead, shift your notion of fun to nonfood activities. You likely have a few favorites that don't involve eating. Build on these until you shift the balance from drinks and dinner to window-shopping or visiting a new art exhibit. If you do want to grab a bite, stick to lunch. It's easier to eat light, and you probably won't order cocktails.

Weekend think: I run around all week; now I just want to kick back.

Healthier splurge: Try a little active relaxation.

Some decompressing is essential, but planting yourself on the couch for hours can lead to trouble. A long stretch of inactivity can inspire compulsive nibbling, especially if boredom is one of your overeating triggers, says Gullo. And the immobility quickly adds up: Skip your regular 1-mile walk, add those extra 222 calories you tend to eat on weekends, and that alone can equal a gain of about 7 pounds a year! Sure, you can indulge in afternoon channel surfing, but not all day long. Impose a time limit; 2 hours is fine. And use that extra time to do something good for yourself, such as chopping veggies for dinner that night and snacks to take to work the next week. Also, don't forget to work downtime into your week so you don't feel as exhausted come the weekend.

Weekend think: A predinner cocktail is par for the course.

Healthier splurge: Drink it during the meal.

With fewer responsibilities and no early morning wake-up calls, even weekday teetotalers don't think twice about a cocktail before dinner—and then another while they eat. The problem: "Alcohol breaks down inhibitions, so it's harder to make healthy food choices when you do sit down," says Gary Foster, PhD, director of the Center for Obesity Research and Education at Temple University. A glass of Cabernet and a few handfuls of mixed nuts while making dinner or waiting to be seated can add up to more than 600 calories, and that's even before the appetizer. Instead, have the wine with your meal, and save added calories by swapping fries for veggies or sharing the lower-cal sorbet, not the chocolate cake. Choose high-quality drinks you'll want to savor, such as vintage wine or single malt scotch, over high-cal fruity concoctions, and sub in one or two club sodas with lime.

> With 3 grams of satisfying fiber, an apple is the perfect on-the-go snack.

Weekend think: I'll just have one last hurrah before I start my diet on Monday.

Healthier splurge: Drop the "last supper" mindset.

Healthy eating doesn't have an on/off switch; it's a way of life, says Dave Grotto, RD, a spokesperson for the American Dietetic Association. He encourages his clients to treat themselves during the week, maybe with a light beer one night or a child's-size ice cream cone another, so they're not feeling deprived and desperate enough to polish off a half-pint of ice cream on Friday night for 500 calories. If you blow it, don't wait until Monday to get back on track; start at your next meal or snack. Besides, giving yourself free rein on the weekend can reactivate negative eating patterns that are bound to carry over into the following week, says Gullo. Keep it up, and extra pounds are almost guaranteed.

Weekend think: Obligations throw off my usual routine.

Healthier splurge: Take control wherever and whenever you can.

Between errands, quality time with the kids, grocery shopping, and household chores, your weekends are often too packed to accommodate your regular diet-and-exercise schedule. But part of developing healthy habits for life is about adapting, says Foster. It just takes a few adjustments: Toss a low-cal energy bar or apple into your bag before hitting the mall so you're not tempted by the food court; if you know you're going to be on the road all afternoon, have a later breakfast; or if restaurant reservations aren't until late, snack on string cheese and whole-grain crackers to hold you over, and then order lean fish or meat and vegetables for dinner. It's okay to shuffle around meals and snacks, just don't skip them or your hunger will overpower you, says Katherine Tallmadge, RD, author of *Diet Simple*. And plan active family outings that aren't doable during the week, such as a tennis match with your spouse or a hike with the kids. You burn slightly more calories than you would at your 9-to-5 desk job, which helps even out a sensible weekend splurge.

chapter 12

THE
DO-IT-YOURSELF DIET

Create an eating plan that's yours and yours alone

Every season brings a new crop of diet books to store shelves. That's not surprising, because more than 60 percent of Americans say they want to lose weight. But what is surprising is that most of us don't stick to these printed plans, according to recent market research. In fact, the most popular—and successful—diet today is the one we make up ourselves.

"The key is to take a few proven weight loss tricks and personalize them," says Lisa Young, PhD, a professor of nutrition at New York University. So rather than adapting your life to fit a set of rules, you adapt the rules to fit your life. Here, we look at popular strategies backed by solid research and offer smart, practical ways to make them work for you.

WHAT WORKS: CUT CARBOHYDRATES

It's simple math, really: The average American eats about twice the recommended daily servings of grains (many in the form of refined flour products such as white bread, pasta,

Outsmart These Diet Traps

Here are our best eating-plan pairings for five of the most common rough spots.

Fancy Dinner Out

The formula = Boost Protein + Volumize

Have a high-protein snack midafternoon (such as almonds and fresh fruit) to take the edge off your hunger. Then order a bowl of broth-based soup or a green salad before the meal.

Overscheduled Day

The formula = Journal + Use Meal Replacements

The night before, try to plan out your day with a reverse food journal (see page 102). Toss a bar or shake and an apple into your bag in case plans change or you're starving with no time to buy lunch.

The 4 p.m. Munchies

The formula = Cut Carbs, Volumize + Boost Protein

Skip hunger-stimulating refined carbs such as sweets and white bread in favor of only whole grains, such as whole wheat crackers. (Pick those that contain at least 3 grams of

and sweets), plus about 20 teaspoons of sugar (mostly from sweetened drinks). Eliminating those nutrient-wimpy simple carbs cuts a big source of empty calories; skipping even just one 20-ounce cola every day saves you 17 teaspoons of sugar, 250 calories—and about 26 pounds over the course of a year!

Do It Your Way

Your body needs carbohydrates for energy; what you should do is eat smaller amounts of healthier ones, says Kathy McManus, RD, director of nutrition at Brigham and Women's Hospital in Boston. Here's how.

fiber per serving.) Bulk up your lunch with extra vegetables, such as grape tomatoes, baby carrots, or red bell pepper strips, and be sure to have a few ounces of protein, such as thin slices of lean ham on whole-grain bread or a chopped egg and a handful of sunflower seeds on a salad.

A Party Buffet

The formula = Boost Protein + Volumize

Fill at least three-quarters of your plate with low-calorie buffet standbys that are rich in fiber, water, or (low-fat) protein, such as shrimp cocktail, vegetables, lean meats, and fruits.

Late-Night Cravings

The formula = Journal + Volumize

Jot down what you eat on every trip to the kitchen. If you must munch while watching TV, choose low-cal foods you can eat more of, such as air-popped popcorn or a plate of cut-up veggies.

Choose whole grains. They're an important source of nutrients and help keep your blood sugar steady between meals and your appetite in check.

Have just one with every meal and snack. That'll get you the appropriate five or six servings a day. To control portions, picture your plate as a clock and limit your carbs to the space between noon and 3 p.m.

Balance the bad carbs. If you do eat refined foods, such as white bread, pair them with a food that has protein or healthy fat, such as hummus. That will help nix a blood sugar spike-and-crash, says Cathy Nonas, RD, director of the Diabetes and Obesity Programs at North General Hospital in New York City.

WHAT WORKS: EAT HIGH-VOLUME FOODS

When you're hungry, you want to eat. Choose foods high in water and fiber and low in calories (think salad and broth-based soup), and you can eat a lot, feel full, and lose weight. Consuming supersize portions activates stretch receptors in your stomach, which then fire off "full" signals to your brain, but you've filled up and stretched without overdoing it on calories.

Do It Your Way

Add heft to every meal by reducing your portion of low-volume foods and folding in high-volume (but low-cal) ones. Fruits and vegetables, which are 80 to 95 percent water, are good additions, as are air-filled foods, such as puffed cereal instead of flat flakes. Here are some more simple swaps to fill your belly faster with more nutrients but far fewer calories.

LOW VOLUME	HIGH VOLUME
Cheese and crackers	6 cups of popcorn sprinkled with Parmesan cheese
Dried fruit and nut mix	Fresh fruit, such as strawberries or grapes, and ¼ cup of nuts
Rice	Half your usual amount cooked with a box of frozen veggies

WHAT WORKS: BOOST PROTEIN

Protein can take about 4 hours to digest, while carbs take only 2; slower digestion means you feel fuller longer. Plus, protein may help jack up your metabolism: In a new study from Purdue University, dieters who ate 30 percent of their calories from protein preserved more lean body mass while losing weight than those who ate only 18 percent. The more lean body mass you hold on to, the more calories you burn at rest.

Do It Your Way

Forget the cheese and bacon of diets past; instead, add a little protein to every meal and snack, says McManus.

Choose healthy sources. That means proteins with unsaturated fats (such as salmon and soy), not the cholesterol-boosting saturated kind (packed into fatty cuts of beef and whole dairy products).

Stick to proper serving sizes. Three ounces of lean meat looks like a deck of cards, the same amount of fish is the size of a checkbook, and your thumb marks an ounce of cheese.

Add protein to your favorites. Combine ground turkey or shrimp with spaghetti and sauce; stir 1 ounce of walnuts into oatmeal; spread a little almond butter on toast before the jam.

WHAT WORKS: REPLACE MEALS WITH BARS AND SHAKES

These products make portion control a snap. "It's calorie cutting without a calculator," says Nonas. An analysis of studies from Columbia University found that women who had one to two liquid meal replacements daily lost an extra 2 pounds per month compared with other dieters who had the same calories.

Do It Your Way

Think of a bar or shake as your go-to food when you're in a pinch. Whether you use them as a meal or as a snack, look for at least 3 grams of fiber, 10 grams of protein, and 3 grams or less saturated fat, and follow these healthy eating guidelines:

As a meal: Most bars and shakes have about 220 calories, so pair either with a small salad with low-fat dressing or a piece of fruit to help fill you up.

As a snack: Between meals, 220 calories is too much. If you have a bar late in the afternoon, for example, cut dinner by half to keep your calorie counts in check.

WHAT WORKS: KEEP A FOOD DIARY

Journaling helps expose bad habits that may otherwise fly under the radar, so you can change them. "When you write down what you eat, you eat less," says Anne Fletcher, RD, author of *Thin for Life*. A study from Kaiser Permanente Center for Health Research showed that keeping a food diary was a better predictor of weight loss than even exercise!

Do It Your Way

Beat journal boredom—and the guilt that comes with committing that cookie to paper—by planning your ideal eating day: Essentially, keep a "reverse" diet diary, where you map out your menu ahead of time and try to stick to it. Track your victories, too: Buy gold star stickers, and put one in your planner for every serving of veggies. "The positive reinforcement builds confidence and motivation, and that's key to success," says McManus.

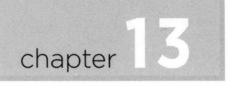
SECRETS OF
THE BIGGEST LOSER
STARS

The stars of the hit TV show reveal their diet strategies, workout hints, and the ab moves that really get results

3 30,000 calories. If you watched the third season of NBC's hit reality show, you'll know that's how many calories contestants Heather and Kai burned on a quest to take back their health—and win $250,000.

The season's over (another contestant, Erik, won, in case you missed it!), but we wanted to take a look back at the challenges these women faced on the show and then look ahead to help them—and those of us who followed along at home—face their ongoing weight-loss challenges. *Prevention* experts provide advice on everything from conquering cravings to carving out exercise time when real-life hassles get in the way.

"I FEEL LIKE I CAN DO ANYTHING!"

Heather Hansen, 36

    Starting weight: 223

    Week 7 weight: 182

    Height: 5'5"

    Starting total cholesterol: 196, dropped to 135

    Blood pressure: 122/80 milligrams of mercury (mm Hg), dropped to 98/70 mm Hg

    Over the past 2 years, Heather went from a size 10 to a size 20 as she juggled the intense demands of work, marriage, and motherhood. She was consuming up to 3,500 calories every day—by her own estimate—but rarely exercised. A vacation to the Bahamas was her wake-up call. "Lying on the beach in your bathing suit at 220-plus pounds is not a situation you want to be in," she says. "I said to myself, I can't live like this. I have to do something."

On the Show

During Heather's audition for *The Biggest Loser*, she jogged in place for hours, raising her knees as high as she could to show the producers, "You can count on me to win!" At the ranch, she paid a price for her competitiveness: a torn calf muscle, bursitis in her knees, and mild tendonitis in her quads. Trainer Kim Lyons guided her toward lower-impact workouts. "If you injure your lower body, there's always something else you can do," Lyons says. "I suggested that Heather try the gentler recumbent bike, elliptical trainer, or rowing machine for a week while she healed."

    Heather's greatest motivation: "It sounds cheesy, but nothing tastes as good as thin feels."

CHALLENGES BACK HOME

Comfort-food cravings. "I'm surrounded by temptation all the time—especially goodies at work. Food is everywhere."

    Prevention Intervention. Make overeating a hassle, not a habit. If Heather's coworkers have to keep snacks around, she should ask them to store goodies in hard-to-reach places, such as a high cabinet or even in a locked closet, says Brian Wansink, PhD, director of the Cornell University Food and Brand Lab and author of *Mindless Eating*. His research found that the farther away you stash appealing food, the less you eat.

Vacation temptations. "On holiday, I look at every single restaurant we pass, with longing," she says.

Prevention **Intervention.** Create a paper trail. To stay mindful of what and how much she's eating, it's key for Heather to keep a food diary, says Cheryl Forberg, RD, the nutritionist for *The Biggest Loser*. In one study, overweight people who kept a food journal for a year lost $41\frac{1}{2}$ pounds, compared with just 17 pounds for those who didn't keep track.

Fitting in fitness. Heather's workout time has dropped 50 percent since she left the ranch. "I plan my workouts around my child's sleep schedule. When I see my fitness equipment, and I see my daughter reading a book, I think, I'd rather be with her. Also, I refuse to exercise on Sundays. I believe in giving the body a day to rest."

Prevention **Intervention.** Merge family and exercise. Lyons suggests that Heather invest in a child's bike seat and helmet so she can cycle with her daughter. Also, fitness strollers are designed for walking and running. "If you walk with your child and do a few lunges, you can burn up to 500 calories an hour," Lyons says.

Heather's Take-It-Off Tips

Plan ahead and indulge wisely. "I used to diet all week and then feel free to eat whatever I wanted on the weekend. Now I just do that on Friday night. But having that meal to look forward to makes it easier to pass on the doughnuts everybody else at the office is eating."

Watch all measures, not just the scales. "Last week, I lost only 1 pound, and I was just incredibly disappointed. But then I got out the measuring tape and learned I lost $3\frac{1}{2}$ inches overall!"

Adjust your social life to fit your goals. "I used to go out to dinner with my friends every month. Now we do outdoor activities—it's fantastic!"

Be patient early on. "Give yourself the chance to lose the first 10 pounds before throwing in the towel. Keep persevering. Because once you pass that benchmark, you get a psychological jump-start and a lot more confidence."

8 Best Belly Busters

The Biggest Loser trainers Bob Harper and Kim Lyons reveal their favorite moves for flattening your abs—no matter what your fitness level.

Beginner

1. Get off balance. "Anytime you're on an unstable surface—and therefore trying to balance—you're developing your core strength. I had my team pull in their guts and stand on one leg while doing bicep curls to help tone their middles."—BH

2. Suck it in. "Very motivated contestants like Adrian wanted to work on their abs even when they weren't working out! One trick: Constantly pull your stomach in to work your transverse abdominis, the deepest layer of muscle in your core. This also improves your posture, so your stomach looks even flatter."—KL

3. Sit and sculpt. "Use a stability ball instead of a chair to work your abs all day long. It's a wonderful way to engage your muscles without having to think about it."—BH

Intermediate

4. Crunch and twist. "Regular crunches are great, especially if you can lift your feet off the ground and make a 90-degree twist from side to side. I recommend three sets of 20—

"I BROKE DOWN MY 'FAT' WALLS"

Kai Hibbard, 28

   Starting weight: 262

   Week 7 weight: 208

   Height: 5'5"

   Starting total cholesterol: 263, dropped to 158

   Blood pressure: 140/91 mm Hg, dropped to 110/78 mm Hg

Kai was an emotional eater who stuffed her feelings with food. After her divorce, she says, "I coped by eating a lot of ice cream and mac and cheese." As she gained, reaching 262 pounds, she gave up the outdoor activities that she loved, such as white water rafting

more if you can. Heather makes these even harder by holding free weights behind her head."—KL

5. Get on the ball. "Do 5 to 8 minutes of crunches on a stability ball to isolate the transverse abdominis and rectus abdominis, the muscles that go straight across and up and down your abs. This is the only ab work that Kai wanted to do!"—KL

6. Ride on. "Do up to 10 minutes of bicycle pedaling in the air while you are lying on your back to work your abdominals."—BH

Advanced

7. Make like a superhero. "Get on your stomach, and lift your arms and legs off the ground like Superman. Then get up into the plank (with your back straight, feet and hands on floor) and lift one arm and the opposite leg like Spiderman—Heather can hold it for over a minute. It works your whole core in a circle."—BH

8. Work your back. "Many people forget that back strength helps support your abs. So do some back extensions on a stability ball. I suggest doing as many back extensions as you can do regular crunches."—KL

and running. "My life became completely circumscribed," she says. "I lost all focus on what I wanted to accomplish physically."

On the Show

Kai's biggest challenges were the long hours of running and the rigorous ab workouts *The Biggest Loser* trainers demanded. "Moving that much body weight was so hard for her," says Lyons. Kai also had to face down her emotional demons. "I learned that I had walls up—literally," she says. "Fat was my way of being invisible." But as she trimmed down, she realized it was time to deal with her difficult emotional issues. "I couldn't live in denial anymore," she says.

Challenges Back Home

A stubborn plateau. "I'm losing and regaining the same 2 pounds even though I am doing everything right."

Prevention **Intervention.** Ramp up your workout. "A plateau means your body is getting used to the exercise you've been doing," says Lyons, so shake up your routine. For example, Kai started gaining weight even though she was running long distances for endurance. But switching to a more demanding activity, such as sprinting, to boost the heart rate and burn more calories could reignite weight loss.

Spending time on the road. Kai is starting law school in Maine. To get there, she and her father are driving all the way from Alaska. "I am going to have to be very careful not to fill those hours with mindless eating," she says.

Prevention **Intervention.** Plan ahead. "Before she goes, she should Google YMCAs and hotel gyms on her route that'll give her a day pass. While her father takes a rest from driving, she can be exercising," says *Prevention* fitness advisor Chris Freytag. Finally, says Stephen Gullo, PhD, author of *The Thin Commandments*, the trick is to avoid being tempted by the burgers and fries. Kai should research restaurant chains that serve lighter fare—and what low-calorie meals are available if the only eatery for miles has a drive-thru window.

Kai's greatest motivation: "Having people care that I get healthy again is my best incentive. Losing weight and learning to let down my defenses has brought me closer to my family and friends."

Kai's Take-It-Off Tips

Learn to love lunges and squats. "I do tons of both. They're the no-excuses moves you can do anywhere, even if you're stuck in an elevator."

Use regret as a tool. "The remorse over a chocolate sundae is going to last a lot longer than the pleasure of eating it."

Mark your progress visually. "Even after I had lost 54 pounds, I couldn't see that I looked different. But when I was able to fit into Heather's much smaller shirt, something clicked, and I was able to see my new shape more clearly."

Ask for tough love. "Remind your family that it's incredibly supportive not to invite you out for a big dinner."

No matter what, don't put it off. "Before, when I overindulged, I used to say, 'I'm definitely going to start my diet Monday.' It never ever worked. Now when I fall off the wagon, I get right back on again."

"I LOST 44 POUNDS AT HOME"

Adrian Kortesmaki, 22

    Starting weight: 227

    Dropped to: 183

    Height: 5'4"

    Starting total cholesterol: 208, went down to 113

While attending the University of North Dakota, this former high school athlete abandoned her healthy habits in favor of late-night partying and a diet of beer and pizza. "Other people gained the freshman 15. I gained a whopping 60 pounds!" she says.

With the Club

Unlike Heather and Kai, contestant Adrian followed a Biggest Loser Club program (www.biggestloserclub.com) at home while also getting advice from show experts. "The first time I went running, I couldn't do more than 2 minutes, so I alternated running, skipping, and walking. Within 2 months, I was running a mile in under 10 minutes."

Challenge at Home

Nights out with friends. "There are people who think I'm no fun because I'm always wanting to eat healthy. Last night, someone even said, 'Please have a beer and pizza.'"

***Prevention* Intervention.** Avoid social eating. The impulse to chow down in groups is so strong, it's mathematically predictable, says Wansink. People who eat with just one person consume 35 percent more, and those who eat with seven or more people consume 96 percent more, a Georgia State University study found. Instead, do another activity where food isn't the focus. Stick to your guns. "Find support at the gym, or get your friends eating better and working out, too," says Freytag. That way, all of you have the same goals.

Adrian's Take-It-Off Tips

Eat a rainbow. "I get my nutrients from all colors of fruits and vegetables—pale foods like chips are never the right fuel."

Don't compare yourself with your formerly fit self. "Pretend you are starting from the beginning. Focus on how fit and healthy you're going to be."

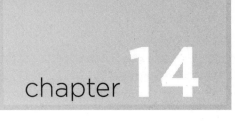

chapter 14

NO-GAIN GUIDE TO VACATION DINING

Stay slim on your next getaway, from all-you-can-eat cruising to fireside camping, how to eat, drink, and not blow your diet

t's your vacation; you've earned the right to indulge. The trick is to not undo all the health gains you've made the rest of the year. Here are simple strategies that let you have your cake, fruity drink, or burger—without gaining an ounce.

IN THE CAR

Driving all day cuts your average daily calorie burn by 400. Follow these tips to help readjust your intake (from your normal 1,800 calories to 1,400, for example) and bypass the thousands of junk-food-filled rest stops along US highways.

Drink up. "The recirculated air in a car can make you thirsty, which you might mistake for hunger," says Charles Stuart Platkin, MPH, founder of www.dietdetective.com. Keep plenty of water on hand.

The Top Places to Stay Fit

We looked at dozens of airports, hotels, and fast-food restaurants to find these healthiest locales.

Leanest Airport

Detroit Metropolitan Wayne County: All but two of this airport's 56 eateries were deemed healthy in a 2006 survey. Top picks for high-fiber, cholesterol-free meals: grilled veggie sandwich at Max & Erma's and sushi and seaweed salad at Musashi. Pack gym clothes for a long layover: $15 buys a day pass to the Westin hotel's gym (terminal A). Find other in-airport workout centers at www.airportgyms.com.

Lowest Cal Drive-Thru

Chick-fil-A: Avoid the breakfast items (too high in fat), but enjoy a healthy offering of salads and sandwiches, such as the Southwest Chargrilled Salad (240 calories, 8 grams fat) and the Chargrilled Chicken Sandwich (270 calories, 3.5 grams fat).

Fittest Hotel Chain

Westin Hotels: You can request an in-room treadmill or stationary bike, plus your pick of Pilates, yoga, and Spinning DVDs. Some US Virgin Island locations offer hula hoop classes set to '50s music, or you can play tennis with a pro on Grand Slam surfaces at the Grand Bahama Island resort. The Chicago Westin even offers freshly laundered workout clothes and sneakers.

Seek fresh food. Although a handful of drive-thrus sit right off the highway, a grocery store—with many more good-for-you options—is probably only a few minutes further. There, you can get a healthy meal—turkey on whole wheat from the deli, an apple, and fat-free yogurt—for less than 350 calories. Or pick up a copy of *Healthy Highways*, a guide to more than 1,900 nutritious eateries across the United States. Download updates at www.healthyhighways.com before you depart, to help you plan your meal stops.

Pack healthy snacks. Load a cooler with low-cal, protein-rich foods, such as apple slices and peanut butter. The protein keeps you fuller longer. Our favorite: Rubbermaid 9-Liter ThermoElectric Travel Cooler and Warmer ($50; Target). For a longer haul, consider renting a car with a built-in cooler, such as the Dodge Caliber or Avenger.

> "I pack running shoes for me and inline skates and a helmet for my daughter, and we head out, wherever we are."
>
> —Kristen Sapienza, 39, Pasadena, Maryland

AT A CAMPSITE

Fresh air, stories around the fire, and dinners under the stars: For most of us, that's the perfect recipe for a weekend in the woods. Here are the right ingredients to make it healthier.

Trade the dogs, swap the s'mores. Instead of all-beef, get turkey, veggie, or tofu hot dogs—all lower in fat. And to shave many calories off dessert, try this tweaked s'mores recipe: Break up a 100-calorie Hershey's Dark chocolate or a Cadbury Thins Premium Dark chocolate bar, and wrap it in foil with one large marshmallow and sliced banana; roast a few minutes over the fire, then grab a spoon.

Make a fish stop. Swing by a grocery store on the way to the grounds for a piece of trout or salmon. (You don't have to catch it—unless you want to.) Season with olive oil, salt, and pepper, and serve with easy-to-prepare dehydrated vegetables. (The site www.harmony housefoods.com has a great selection.) For simple outdoor grilling, get the Coleman Fold 'n' Go Propane InstaStart Stove ($80, fuel sold separately; available at sporting goods stores). With two separate skillets, you can make the fish in one and veggies in the other.

Fuel up for hikes, snack lightly for strolls. Pack some sustenance if you're heading out for 2- or 3-mile stretches. Easy-to-tote fruit-and-nut bars, such as Larabar (starting at 190 calories, 9 grams fat) or Clif Nectar (starting at 150 calories, 5 grams fat), provide the energy you need, and you'll burn off the calories. For less strenuous exercise, stick to fruit or a few almonds.

ON A CRUISE

> "Every year, I go camping with a group of friends, and we divvy up cooking. Each person makes one day's worth of low-fat and low-carb meals and snacks. This way, we know we're eating well, and we get to try different menus."
>
> —Patricia Davis, 58, Micanopy, Florida

With pizza served at 3 p.m., dinner at 6 p.m., and a 24-hour dessert cart, most cruises are one big, endless buffet. "Just because they feed you 18 times a day doesn't mean you have to eat 18 times a day," says Davida F. Kruger, MSN, author of *The Diabetes Travel Guide*. Try to follow your at-home eating schedule, as well as the following tips.

Rein in the rum runners. Enjoy your favorite fruity concoction with lunch, or a glass of wine with dinner, but when you're lounging by the pool, strolling the deck, or playing a midnight game of poker, order an alcohol-free fruit smoothie in a 5-ounce martini glass for about 90 calories, or a seltzer spiked with juice and lime for around 30.

Scan the menus. Several cruise lines provide meals low in calories and fat: Cunard's Queen Mary 2 offers gourmet options prepared by Canyon Ranch Spa chefs, including

Drink and Still Drop Pounds

Try these three new, ice-cold, low-cal treats for the road.

Jamba Juice Peach Perfection Smoothie: A blend of peaches, mangoes, and strawberries, it provides three servings of fruit, as well as 4 grams of fiber. (200 calories, 0 grams fat)

Starbucks Orange Crème Frappuccino Light: This combo of cream and zesty orange juice has half the calories of the full-fat version. (110 calories, 0 grams fat)

Seattle's Best Coffee Cold-Brewed Vanilla Latte: Get a caffeine fix with this mix of iced coffee, vanilla syrup, and milk (ask for fat-free). Prefer soy milk or sugar-free syrup? It's fully customizable. (80 calories, 0 grams fat)

Mightier Than the Syringe?

If you travel a lot, consider taking along an insulin pen instead of a syringe. Like syringes, pens use a needle to inject insulin into the body, but they make the process go a little quicker because the insulin comes in prefilled cartridges.

You can choose from disposable or refillable pens, and cartridges come in a variety of dosages to meet individual needs. Some varieties have a dosage knob for setting the amount. Insulin pens can make life easier for people on a multidose regimen, people who have trouble filling syringes (such as those with arthritis in their hands), and folks who are constantly on the go. Talk with your doctor.

tortilla soup with pico de gallo (85 calories, 5 grams fat) and spinach and roasted beet salad (110 calories, 4 grams fat). Crystal Cruises has low-carb ice cream, and Silversea Cruises offers Iced Key Lime Cheesecake and Peach Crumb Cobbler at less than 200 calories each.

Always use the salad plate. Be it for the breakfast bar, lunch buffet, or dinner entrée, this tried-and-true trick will help keep your portions in control. Use it to eat a salad before each meal, too—another way to cut your total calories.

"I do a mini-workout every morning—even when I'm out of town. It prevents me from drinking too much at night, because I know exercising with even a teeny hangover is no fun at all."

—Nina McCollum, 38, Cleveland

chapter 15

DIET ROADBLOCKS

Avoid the 10 surprising reasons that you aren't losing
weight when you should be

f losing weight were simple, Spanx would be just a screen name in an S&M chat room. But dieting is complicated: You can even screw up without realizing it. For instance, who would ever think that working out in the morning or cranking up the AC might be the reason you're not slimming down? Luckily, once you've identified these flubs, fixing them is a cinch.

ROADBLOCK #1: YOU WORK OUT AT 6 A.M.

What's wrong with that? Morning workouts are great—if you go to bed at 10 p.m. In a recent study in the *American Journal of Epidemiology*, people who slept 7 or more hours a night were less likely to put on weight than people who didn't. Those who slept only 6 hours a night were 12 percent more likely to gain substantial weight—33 pounds on average over the course of 16 years! (People who slept a measly 5 hours had a 32 percent chance of gaining 30 or more pounds.) Other studies have linked lack of sleep to a higher body mass index (BMI) and have found that it negatively affects levels of the appetite-regulating hormones ghrelin and leptin.

Detour: Don't sacrifice your snooze time—not even for an extra-long run. And quality matters more than quantity, so taking a siesta later won't help. "In a 20-minute power nap, you don't get into the deep-sleep stage," says Donna Taliaferro, PhD, associate professor of nursing at the University of Missouri-St. Louis, who conducts research on sleep and circadian rhythms. "You need to go through the cycles of sleep over a few hours to get the restorative rest that allows your body to work properly." Bottom line: You're better off sleeping through your workout every other day than stumbling to a sunrise run on too few z's.

ROADBLOCK #2: YOU'RE A TEETOTALER (OR A SOT!)

What's wrong with that? Alcohol may not be the diet kryptonite you thought it was. Recent research showed that those who have a single drink a couple times a week have a lower risk of becoming obese than either teetotalers or heavy drinkers. Those who consume more than four drinks daily, on the other hand, boost their odds of obesity by 46 percent.

Detour: Go ahead and have a drink; just avoid belly-busters such as a 245-calorie piña colada. Instead, raise a glass of heart-smart Merlot (123 calories per 5 ounces), Bud Light (110 calories per 12 ounces), champagne (88 calories per 4 ounces), or sake (39 calories per ounce). Or mix a 100-calorie cocktail, such as vodka and diet tonic, or tequila and club soda. "Just make sure you drink it with some healthy food, such as raw veggies with low-fat dip or whole wheat pita and hummus," advises Dawn Jackson Blatner, RD, a spokesperson for the American Dietetic Association. Eating slows the rise of alcohol in your blood—which cuts the odds you'll order the deep-fried mozzarella sticks.

ROADBLOCK #3: YOU CRANK UP THE AC

What's wrong with that? Al Gore wants you to lay off the thermostat to save the planet. Here's how it can save (the shape of) your own behind, too: In a study published in *Physiology & Behavior*, researchers found that exposure to temperatures above the "thermoneutral zone"—the artificial climate we create with clothes, heating, or air conditioning—decreases our appetite and food intake. "At a slightly uncomfortable 81 degrees, the people in the study experienced a 20 percent decrease in appetite and ate 10 percent less than at 72 degrees," says lead author Margriet S. Westerterp-Plantenga, PhD, a professor of food-intake regulation in the department of human biology at Maastricht University in the Netherlands.

Detour: Instead of cranking up the air conditioner every time you feel a little warm, learn to endure or adjust to slightly warmer conditions. Hitting the "off" button is well worth a little discomfort if it helps you lose the saddlebags or spare tire.

ROADBLOCK #4: YOU LOG EXTRA MILES ON THE TREADMILL TO MAKE UP FOR GIANT MEALS

What's wrong with that? When it comes to dieting, success isn't 90 percent perspiration. You can't achieve lasting weight loss via exercise alone. But a new study in the *Journal of Clinical Endocrinology and Metabolism* found that dieting can shrink your fat zones just as effectively as dieting plus exercise.

Detour: If you try the diet-only approach, you need a clear idea of how much you should be eating. Multiply your weight by 10, then add your weight again to that sum: That gives you the number of calories you need for maintaining your current weight without activity. For example, 135 pounds x 10 = 1,350 + 135 = 1,485 calories. Eat more than that regularly, and your "loose-fit" pants won't anymore; eat less, and your muffin top will start melting away. But not so fast—before you burn your gym membership, read on about sarcopenia.

ROADBLOCK #5: YOU IGNORE SARCOPENIA

What's wrong with that? Sarcopenia, in case you weren't paying attention to your medical TV dramas, is age-related muscle loss, and it can start in your 30s. If you don't take action now, you could begin to lose as much as 1 to 2 percent of your muscle mass by the time you hit 50. Less muscle means you burn fewer calories and store more of them as fat.

Detour: The key to stopping muscle meltdown is to strengthen your back, shoulders, arms, and thighs. "When you increase lean muscle mass, you burn more calories, even when you're sitting down doing nothing," says Amy Campbell, MS, RD, education program manager for health care services at the Joslin Diabetes Center of the Harvard Medical School. Try the strength circuit beginning on page 167 and start sculpting at least twice a week. And keep it up after you reach your goal weight: Studies show that if you don't exercise regularly (60 minutes of moderate physical activity a day), the pounds can creep back on.

ROADBLOCK #6: YOU'RE SHOOTING FOR A REALISTIC SIZE INSTEAD OF A NEAR-IMPOSSIBLE ONE

What's wrong with that? According to a study of 1,801 people, published in the *International Journal of Obesity*, women, in particular, who set unrealistically high weight-loss goals dropped more weight in 24 months than those who kept their expectations low.

Detour: The study authors concluded that having an optimistic goal motivated women to lose more weight. And the participants who failed to reach their magic number did not quit trying to drop the weight. Could aiming for Sienna Miller's figure really help you reach your goal weight healthfully? "If you're a driven person, and a lofty goal motivates you," says Blatner, "it can work."

ROADBLOCK #7: YOU'VE BEEN POPPING M&M'S LIKE THEY'RE ADVIL

What's wrong with that? You've heard the news: Cocoa can lower blood pressure; reduce the risk of heart attack, stroke, diabetes, and dementia; and possibly even prevent cancer. But the research isn't as delicious as it seems. The cocoa bean products used in the studies are a far cry from the highly processed chocolate candy you find on the shelves of your local store. "Milk chocolate contains about 150 calories and 10 grams of fat per ounce," says Campbell.

Detour: The key here is small doses. Dark chocolate, which retains more of the bean during processing, generally has slightly less fat and fewer calories than milk chocolate has—plus, it's richer, so less goes a longer way. We like CocoaVia's Crispy Chocolate Bar (90 calories, 5 grams fat) or Hershey's Special Dark Chocolate Stick (60 calories, 3.5 grams fat). If dark doesn't do it for you, opt for low-cal choices such as a half cup of Breyers French Chocolate Double Churn Fat-Free Ice Cream (90 calories, 0 grams fat).

ROADBLOCK #8: YOU THINK "WATER-RICH DIET" MEANS MORE TRIPS TO THE COOLER

What's wrong with that? Water in your glass is good, but water in your food can have serious slimming power. In a new *American Journal of Clinical Nutrition* study, obese people ages 20 to 60 were told to either reduce their fat intake or increase their intake of water-rich foods, such as fruits and veggies. Although they ate more, the people in the water-rich group chose foods that were more filling—yet had fewer calories—so they still lost 33 percent more weight in the first 6 months than did the people in the reduced-fat group.

Detour: Fill up on food that's high in water. Some good choices in addition to fruits and veggies: broth-based, low-sodium soups; oatmeal and other whole grains; and beans. For other filling options, consult *The Volumetrics Eating Plan: Techniques and Recipes for Feeling Full on Fewer Calories*, by Barbara Rolls, PhD.

ROADBLOCK #9: YOU GIVE UP JUNK FOOD TODAY BUT PUT OFF JOINING A GYM

What's wrong with that? Tackling one goal at a time is supposed to help you succeed. But new research published in the *Archives of Internal Medicine* bucks that conventional wisdom. In a study of more than 200 people who smoked, had high blood pressure, and weren't extremely active, one group was asked to quit the butts, cut back on dietary sodium, and increase physical activity all at once. Another group addressed one bad habit at a time. The group that tackled all their problems simultaneously had the higher success rate after 18 months.

Detour: Combining your goals may work for the same reason job negotiations do:

When you ask for everything, you're more likely to get something. Put this thinking to the test by creating a healthy eating and exercise plan and throwing all your energy into following both.

ROADBLOCK #10: YOU NEVER THINK ABOUT POTASSIUM

What's wrong with that? A recent Canadian study concluded that getting more potassium might help lower your weight and blood pressure. Levels measured in study participants were proportional to their diet and weight. "That makes sense," says Blatner. "The richest sources of potassium are beans, vegetables, and fruit, so the person with high potassium levels is consuming a lot of these foods, which are low in calories and are the most filling."

Detour: You should aim for 4,700 milligrams of potassium each day. Supplements may help you hit that target, but doctors don't recommend them for everyone. Try filling up on white beans (1 cup: 1,000 milligrams potassium), winter squash (1 cup: 494 milligrams), spinach (1 cup: 840 milligrams), baked potato with skin (926 milligrams), yogurt (1 cup: 600 milligrams), halibut (4 ounces: 566 milligrams), and orange juice (1 cup: 473 milligrams).

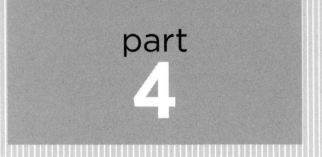

part
4

MOVE IT

medical
BREAKTHROUGHS

Want the latest exercise news? Look no further!

MAKE SMALL CHANGES, GET BIG GAINS

You don't need an extreme lifestyle makeover to reduce your risk of diabetes. Researchers in the United Kingdom wanted to determine the association between exercise, fitness, and something they call "metabolic risk," which includes your waist size, blood sugar level, cholesterol levels, and blood pressure, all of which are predictive of your diabetes risk.

For 1 year, the researchers studied 365 adults with family histories of diabetes and discovered that small increases in activity and fitness were associated with a reduction of metabolic risk. They hope that further research to determine how this relates specifically to reducing the risk of diabetes will help provide better preventive measures for diabetes in the future.

DON'T DITCH THOSE DUMBBELLS

Combining cardio and weights controls blood sugar levels better than either activity alone, reports a study in the journal *Annals of Internal Medicine*. Adults with type 2 diabetes who did 45 minutes of each activity three times weekly lowered their blood sugar levels further than those who did 45 minutes of either cardio or weight training. After 22 weeks, their levels had dropped 0.97 percent (equal to a 15 percent reduction in heart attack or stroke risk), compared with 0.5 percent in the monoexercisers.

Why? Cardio burns glucose (sugar) for energy, while lifting increases the demand for energy by upping muscle mass, leaving less sugar in the blood, says lead author Ronald Sigal, MD, MPH. Don't have 90 minutes to spare? Thirty minutes of each can do the same trick.

SWEAT THE SMALL STUFF

Don't dread those dirty dishes: Low-intensity activities can decrease diabetes and cardiovascular disease risk, reports a *Diabetes Care* study. Researchers found that spending more than 8 hours a day on sedentary activities, such as sitting at a desk, raised subjects' blood sugar 3 percent. But spending about 6 hours a day doing light activities, such as washing dishes, lowered levels 3 percent. Research has shown that a sustained blood sugar increase of 13 percent ups the risk of cardiovascular death by 9 percent. Minor moves could keep you out of the danger zone, researchers say. Desk-bound? Swap your chair for a fitness ball to work your core.

TIME IT RIGHT

It's challenging to fit exercise into an overly scheduled day. Wouldn't it be great to know the time of day that fitting exercise in would give you the most

Percentage decrease in your risk for diabetes if you walk briskly for 35 minutes every day, according to Harvard researchers reporting in the journal *Diabetes Care*: 30 percent

insulin control bang for your exercise buck? That's what researchers at the Research Center for Exercise and Health in Leuven, Belgium, thought. They studied seven sedentary men with metabolic syndrome, which is a group of risk factors that put a person at risk for diabetes. Some of the men exercised before breakfast, others exercised after breakfast, and still others didn't exercise at all. The researchers checked their blood sugar and blood fat levels throughout the day.

The researchers discovered that the men burned fat more quickly when they exercised before breakfast compared with when they exercised after breakfast. But on the other hand, the men's blood sugar levels didn't rise as much when they exercised *after* breakfast as when they had exercised *before* breakfast. And neither exercising before nor after breakfast affected how the men's blood sugar levels were regulated later in the day.

So perhaps if you're trying to burn fat, exercise before breakfast, but if you're looking to keep your blood sugar more stable, exercise after breakfast instead.

SAVE TIME AND TONE YOUR BEHIND

The number of minutes per day of stairclimbing proven to improve heart health: 11 minutes

Stairs or elevator? To save time and boost fitness, climb rather than ride. It shaves off 20 seconds per flight, report University of South Carolina at Aiken researchers who clocked office workers traveling from floor to floor. Plus, stairclimbing burns 100 calories every 11 minutes—as many as jogging—while toning hamstrings, quads, and glutes (the muscles of the hips and thighs), making it one of the best butt firmers around. Not bad for a workday workout.

SET YOUR SIGHTS ON BLASTING FAT

It may sound simple, but it works: For faster toning, target your primary trouble zone first. You get the best results from exercise while your body's still fresh, suggests a study published in the *Journal of Strength and Conditioning Research*. The old thinking was to work large muscle groups (legs, butt) before smaller ones (abs, arms), but fatigue caused people in the study to complete fewer reps at the end of their workouts. Bottom line: For a toned tummy, lead off with abs. Want a better butt in jeans? Start with squats.

WALK OFF 15 PERCENT MORE CALORIES

To lose pounds faster, focus on your arms with every stride, which research has shown can speed your calorie burn. Try these strategies from Mark Fenton, walking expert and author of *The Complete Guide to Walking for Health, Weight Loss, and Fitness.*

Bend your arms to 90 degrees. This makes the swing quick and compact; your feet have no choice but to keep up!

Trace an arc from your waist to your chest as you swing. "Your thumb should brush against your waistband as your elbow goes backward," Fenton says. This move ensures that your arms propel you forward, not flail aimlessly.

Keep your elbows in, and don't let your hands cross past the middle of your chest (in front of your sternum). Too much side-to-side motion drags down your pace.

TAKE THE FAST TRACK TO FITNESS

Here's more evidence that your relationship can boost your health: Older women who rarely miss a workout are three times as likely to have active spouses as those who exercised less consistently (fewer than 25 minutes daily), finds a University of Pittsburgh study. Keep each other on track by scheduling joint workouts, making a weekend hiking date, or training together for a 5K race. Bonus: Exercise enhances your sex life by improving bloodflow and releasing mood-boosting endorphins.

The percentage of couples who stuck with a fitness program when they did it together, according to the *Journal of Sports Medicine and Physical Fitness*: 94 percent

LOVE YOUR WORKOUT

Exercising with people your own age may help you stick with it, suggests a new University of British Columbia survey. Researchers found that of the nearly 1,000 respondents, women of all ages strongly preferred to work out with peers. Numerous studies prove you're more likely to make exercise a habit if you enjoy it, so check out the following Web sites to meet your match.

www.eons.com: Log on to the fitness section of this social networking site (think MySpace.com for grown-ups) to find users looking to partner and share tips.

www.walkstyles.com: Search for a local walking club or workout pal based on your age preference and schedule.

www.prevention.com: Click on Find a Walking Buddy at www.prevention.com/walking and get connected with nearby walkers through our message boards.

TAKE TWENTY

Try this move: The Lounge. Chilling in the middle of a workout can burn more fat than exercising continuously, reports a *Journal of Applied Physiology* study. Scientists measured fat metabolism in seven men as they took three tests: pedaling on a stationary bike for 60 minutes; pedaling for 30, sitting for 20, and then pedaling again for 30; and sitting for 60 minutes. Subjects who took a break had three times the free fatty acids (compounds released when stored fat is used) at the 50-minute mark. During a break, the body may redirect its excess energy into burning fat—so pausing revs up the fat-burning process twice.

Not into time-outs? Interrupt cardio or weight sessions with easy spinning, stretching, or walking.

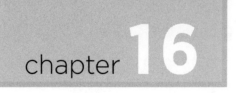

chapter **16**

THE FITNESS FORMULA

Keep your heart healthy, your bones strong, your mind sharp, and your skin glowing and wrinkle-free with our ultimate exercise plan

There really is a fountain of youth: It's called exercise. How? Let us count the ways: In study after study, regular workouts have been proven to insulate you from diabetes, heart disease, cancer, Alzheimer's disease, and stroke. Exercise lowers blood pressure, reduces body fat, raises high-density lipoprotein (HDL) cholesterol (the "good" cholesterol), lowers low-density lipoprotein (LDL) cholesterol (the "bad" cholesterol), improves bloodflow, keeps intestines and the colon healthy, and regulates key hormones.

To ensure you reap all these benefits, we asked leading experts on aging and exercise to devise the ultimate antiaging workout. All agreed that it should include the four cornerstones of age prevention: consistent cardio, intense intervals, weight training, and yoga. Start now, and you can turn back the clock . . . for life.

Your Ultimate 7-Day Plan

This routine combines everything into one easy-to-follow schedule.

Day 1
30 minutes cardio
30 minutes yoga

Day 2
45 minutes intervals/cardio

Day 3
20 minutes weight training
30 minutes yoga

Day 4
30 minutes cardio
30 minutes yoga

Day 5
45 minutes intervals/cardio
20 minutes weight training

Day 6
30 minutes cardio
30 minutes yoga

Day 7
Rest

CONSISTENT CARDIO

The verdict is in: People who exercise almost daily really do keep ticking longer. When scientists pored over data from the famous Framingham Heart Study of more than 5,000 women and men, they discovered that active folks lived nearly 4 years longer than their inactive peers, largely because they sidestep heart disease—the nation's leading killer. Aerobic exercise such as walking, biking, jogging, and swimming protects your heart by lowering blood pressure, reducing "bad" cholesterol, and keeping arteries flexible to improve bloodflow.

Your Rx: 30 minutes, 5 days a week of moderate-intensity aerobic exercise. Work at a pace that allows you to talk freely. If you can sing, you're not exercising hard enough.

To get started, choose an activity you enjoy and do 10 minutes, 5 days a week. Then, increase by 5 minutes each week until you're doing 30 minutes at a time. Dividing your exercise into three 10-minute bouts throughout the day works, too.

More Ways Exercise Keeps You Young

Still not convinced? Read on!

It boosts your mood: Cardio workouts raise levels of the brain's feel-good neurotransmitters like serotonin and norepinephrine.

It helps you sleep: The rhythmic breathing and relaxation of yoga and tai chi help you fall asleep and snooze longer.

It keeps you slim: Beyond burning calories, exercise may also help regulate the production of leptin, the "fat hormone" that controls appetite.

It firms you up: Lifting weights builds muscle—the magic tissue needed to counteract gravity and prevent sagging.

It charges up your sex life: Hormonal changes as you age can lower libido, but just 20 minutes of exercise gets you in the mood by increasing bloodflow to the genitals.

INTENSE INTERVALS

Exercise keeps your mind fit by bringing more blood and oxygen to the noggin, rejuvenating your brain in the process. "The hippocampus, the main area of the brain where memory resides, is particularly susceptible to damage from low bloodflow or lack of oxygen—both of which become more likely as we age," says brain researcher Eric B. Larson, MD, of the Group Health Cooperative in Seattle. Doing bursts of higher-intensity activity will increase bloodflow and oxygen even more.

Your Rx: 45 minutes, twice a week (moderate-paced cardio exercise interspersed with 1-minute speed bursts every 2 minutes). Based on a 1-to-10 scale, you should feel like you're working at an intensity of 7 or 8 (brisk enough that you can talk, but you'd rather not) during the speed bursts and an intensity of 5 or 6 (moderate enough that you can talk freely) the rest of the time.

If you're just starting out, do 15-second intervals, slowly building up to 1 minute as your endurance increases. Because this is cardio exercise, you don't have to do these workouts on top of the steady-paced cardio session on page 135 (although you can if you have the time, and you'll shape up even faster). Just extend two of those workouts and make them intervals.

WEIGHT TRAINING

A healthy heart is key, but unless you have strong bones and muscles, getting up off the couch, climbing the stairs, and walking out the door to enjoy life won't be so easy. Lifting weights is one of the best ways to keep these body systems in tip-top shape, says Wendy Kohrt, PhD, a professor in the division of geriatric medicine at the University of Colorado Health Sciences Center in Denver. And it can help you stand tall—a quick way to look younger.

Your Rx: 20 minutes, twice a week. Pick up two sets of dumbbells (3 and 5 pounds for beginners; 5 and 10 or 10 and 20 if you need an even bigger challenge), available at most department stores or sporting goods stores. Then, follow the strength-building workouts at www.prevention.com/firmbody.

Blister-Battling Socks

For people with diabetes, even minor foot injuries take longer to heal, because diabetes can affect the nerves and circulation in the feet. That's why it's smart to ditch those soggy, chafing cotton socks and graduate to a high-performance pair that stays comfortable mile after mile. In general, people with diabetes should look for socks with minimal seams (which can rub you the wrong way) and extra padding (to provide added protection). Socks shouldn't be too tight, because you don't want to cut off circulation. Also look for ones that are made with fabric that wicks away excess moisture, such as CoolMax.

Shoe-Shopping Strategies

Diabetes can lead to nerve damage to the feet, which can make it tough for you to feel if you're developing a blister or sore spot. To protect your feet—whatever your favorite sport—you should always wear shoes that fit well and don't rub or chafe. When buying shoes:

Try them on at the end of the day, when feet are their largest.

Wear your walking socks. Some styles are really thick, and you may need to go half a size larger with your shoes to accommodate them.

Check inside to make sure there are no seams or bumps that could irritate your feet.

Make sure there's plenty of room—at least a finger's width beyond the end of your longest toe (usually the big toe).

Measure when you're standing up rather than sitting down.

If you just can't find a pair of off-the-shelf shoes that fit comfortably, ask your doctor or podiatrist about Medicare coverage for custom-made shoes or inserts.

YOGA

The less tense you are, the fewer lines and wrinkles you'll develop. One of the best workouts to fight stress? Yoga. In a German study, 3 hours of practice a week lowered the anxiety levels of 16 women ages 26 to 51 by a whopping 30 percent. "As your mouth, jaw, and brows relax, you can literally see the creases soften," says Larry Payne, PhD, director of the Yoga Therapy Rx program at Loyola Marymount University. It may also protect against free radicals, compounds that break down skin's elasticity.

Your Rx: 30 minutes, four times a week. To get started, go to www.prevention.com/youthfulyoga.

chapter 17

THE ULTIMATE WALKING WORKOUT

Lower your blood sugar by walking

Here's something you should know about diabetes: Even if you already have it, you can control the disease and avoid many of its consequences.

The best way to do that is to combine a healthy diet and regular physical activity such as walking. This can help you slim down, which is an important benefit, because being overweight is a major risk factor for diabetes.

But here's some even better news: Walking fights diabetes in ways other than weight loss. Studies are just starting to show the preventive power of fitness. For example, the famous Nurses' Health Study found that women who worked up a sweat more than once a week reduced their risk of developing diabetes by 30 percent. And researchers in China determined that people with high blood sugar who engaged in moderate exercise and made other lifestyle changes were 40 percent less likely to develop full-blown diabetes. It wasn't even vigorous exercise.

The bottom line is: Walking works wonders.

MAKE WALKS WORK FOR YOU

Why does walking have such protective effects? Besides helping you get rid of extra pounds, it actually increases the number of insulin receptors on your cells. Insulin helps blood sugar move into cells, where it needs to go. Otherwise, it just sloshes around in your bloodstream, gumming up the blood vessel walls.

If you've already been diagnosed with diabetes, regular walking can help control the progression of the disease. People who take insulin may be able to reduce the amount of medication they need, because physical activity enables their body to use insulin more efficiently.

As a bonus, walking regularly can help boost your brainpower. Scientists have observed that older people with diabetes sometimes have problems thinking clearly. In one study, physical activity appeared to stimulate just the type of brain activity that had become impaired. Exactly what it is about physical activity that revs up the brain hasn't been determined. But some experts theorize that exercise-related brain activity could be part of the reason why some folks say they are better able to solve sticky problems while they are working out.

Before you begin a walking program, check with your doctor, especially if you already have diabetes. He or she can tell you whether you need to take any special precautions when you work out.

According to diabetes experts, you must exercise for at least 30 minutes, three times a week to enhance your body's use of insulin. If your goal is to lose weight, however, you would do well to walk five to seven times each week. But, of course, you will want to work

Caution

People with diabetes often have difficulty feeling foot problems because of nerve damage associated with the condition. They're also more prone to infection.

To keep your feet healthy, inspect them daily and apply baby powder to keep them dry and to discourage the formation of blisters. If you notice any irritation, consult a physician within 24 hours.

up to that level slowly, especially if you have been sedentary. If you skip a day, don't try to make up for it by walking twice as fast or twice as far during your next workout. Vigorous exercise can actually cause blood sugar to rise, especially in people who have insulin deficiencies.

If you have diabetes, the timing of your walks can help regulate your blood sugar level. People with type 2 (non-insulin-dependent) diabetes may benefit from exercising before meals, which helps control appetite and promote weight loss. For those with type 1 (insulin-dependent) diabetes, it's best not to exercise on an empty stomach. These folks should plan their walks for about an hour or so after a meal, when blood sugar levels are at their highest.

Sometimes, exercise can send blood sugar plummeting. This reaction is most common among people who use insulin. Ask your doctor how much exercise you can tolerate before you need to replenish your store of carbohydrates. And carry a healthy snack— such as a piece of fresh fruit, dried fruit, or some peanuts or trail mix—with you for just this purpose.

Ready, Set, Go!

Here are the pace and exertion levels for all the workouts.

PACE	SPEED (MPH)	HOW IT FEELS	INTENSITY LEVEL*
Warmup, cooldown	2.5	Like window-shopping	3–4
Easy walk	3.0	Easy enough that you can sing	4–5
Brisk walk	3.5	You can talk freely, but no more singing	5–6
Strong walk	4.0	You're slightly breathless	6–7
Power walk	4.5	You can talk in brief phrases, but you'd rather not	7–8
Speed walk	5.0	No breath for chatting!	8–9

*Based on a 1–10 scale, with 1 equivalent to sitting on the sofa and 10 equivalent to sprinting.

THREE WAYS TO WALK OFF WEIGHT

Walking is a great tool for weight management. To get the best results, you need to be consistent, so a routine that fits your lifestyle is key. That's why we developed the perfect 20-, 45-, and 60-minute workouts. Now you can burn calories, tone your body, and boost your energy in whatever time you have.

Another bonus: In a recent study of people with diabetes, those who walked regularly (45 minutes or more, three times a week) showed improvements in their blood pressure and cholesterol levels as well as their body mass index. Just mix and match all three of these workouts on most days, and you can lose up to 3 pounds this month.

Great Reasons to Get Moving

On days when you're having a little trouble getting motivated, glance at this handy reminder of all the good that exercise can do for you! Exercise . . .

Can help control my blood sugar.

Helps insulin work better in my body.

Improves my mood and lowers my stress level.

Can help keep my blood pressure and cholesterol in the healthy range.

Reduces my risk for heart disease and stroke.

Improves my circulation.

Strengthens my muscles and bones.

Keeps my joints flexible.

Can help me achieve and maintain a healthy weight.

Helps me feel better about myself.

Walk 1

In 20 minutes: Boost your energy

No time for a long walk? Then go for speed. You'll burn about 25 percent more calories for every 0.5-mph increase, which is what each new level in the first 10 minutes of the following plan does. "This burns as much fat as possible in a short workout," says certified trainer Debbie Rocker, who designed these workouts. And getting your heart rate up will give you an energy boost that will last all day.

YOUR PLAN AT A GLANCE

TIME	PACE*	INTENSITY LEVEL**
Start	Warmup	3–4
1:00	Easy walk	4–5
3:00	Brisk walk	5–6
5:00	Strong walk	6–7
7:00	Power walk	7–8
9:00	Speed walk	8–9
11:00	Power walk	7–8
13:00	Strong walk	6–7
15:00	Brisk walk	5–6
17:00	Easy walk	4–5
19:00	Cooldown	3–4
20:00	Finish	

*See "Ready, Set, Go" on page 137 for all pace descriptions.

**Based on a 1–10 scale with 1 equivalent to sitting on the sofa and 10 equivalent to sprinting.

Walk 2

In 45 minutes: Sculpt every inch

Shape your arms and tone your abs while you walk off fat with this double-duty workout. By interspersing 2-minute bouts of strength-training, you'll build lean muscle, which keeps your metabolism revved even when you're not exercising. You'll also be doing your heart good. Researchers in Northern Ireland found that women in their 30s and 40s who walked for 45 minutes just twice a week reduced their systolic blood pressure by 5 points in 8 weeks, lowering their risk of stroke and heart attack.

YOUR PLAN AT A GLANCE

TIME	PACE*	INTENSITY LEVEL**
Start	Warmup	3–4
4:00	Strong walk	6–7
7:00	Walking lunges with 10-second break in the middle	
9:00	Strong walk	6–7
12:00	Tree sit, hold 20 seconds, rest 5 seconds, repeat	
14:00	Strong walk	6–7
17:00	Double lift, 3 sets of 10 reps per side, rest 10 seconds between sets	
19:00	Strong walk	6–7
22:00	Reverse curl, 3 sets of 10 reps, rest 10 seconds between sets	
24:00	Strong walk	6–7
27:00	Triceps dip, 2 sets of 10 reps, rest 10 seconds between sets	
29:00	Strong walk	6–7
32:00	Pushup, 2 sets of 10 reps, rest 10 seconds between sets	
34:00	Strong walk	6–7
37:00	Walking lunges with 10-second break in the middle	
39:00	Strong walk	6–7
42:00	Cooldown	3–4
45:00	Finish	

*See exercise descriptions beginning on the opposite page. See "Ready, Set, Go" on page 137 for all pace descriptions.

**Based on a 1–10 scale, with 1 equivalent to sitting on the sofa and 10 equivalent to sprinting.

WALKING LUNGE

TONES BUTT AND LEGS

Stand with your feet together and your hands on your hips. Step forward with your left foot as far as comfortable. Land on your heel, controlling your descent as you bend your knees and drop your hips, keeping your left knee directly above your ankle. Don't lean forward. Stop when your left thigh is parallel to the ground. Stand back up by squeezing your glutes and pushing off with your back toes; bring your right foot next to your left foot. Repeat with your right leg, slowly lowering into a lunge.

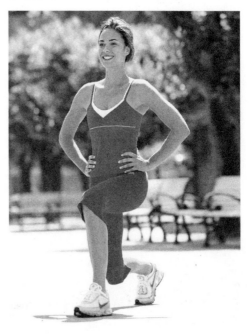

Pain in the Shins

If your shins give you pain at night, it could be because of where you're exercising, or it could be a symptom of something more serious, such as diabetic neuropathy (nerve damage caused by diabetes) or a stress fracture. Walking, jogging, or running on a hard surface can put too much strain on the muscle and bone of your lower legs, causing shin splints. Often, the pain doesn't kick in until hours after you're done exercising. It can even wake you at night. See your doctor to find out if the cause is shin splints or if it's another malady.

If you do have shin splints, take it easy for at least a week, advises Karaanne Gregory, an exercise physiologist at Joslin Diabetes Center in Boston. And strengthen the muscles in the fronts of your lower legs, which will help you sidestep a recurrence.

Here's an easy move: While standing, lift your toes toward your shins 20 times; work up to three sets. When you're ready to resume exercising, wear supportive sneakers that fit well, and try a softer surface, such as an indoor track, to reduce stress on your legs. Afterward, ice your shins for 10 to 15 minutes, and stretch your calf muscles to head off soreness.

TREE SIT

TONES BUTT AND LEGS

Sit with your back against a tree trunk, fence, or wall so your knees are bent at 90 degrees and your ankles are directly beneath your knees. (You can use your hands to help get into position, or if the surface is smooth, slide down into position.) Hold for 20 seconds, then return to the standing position.

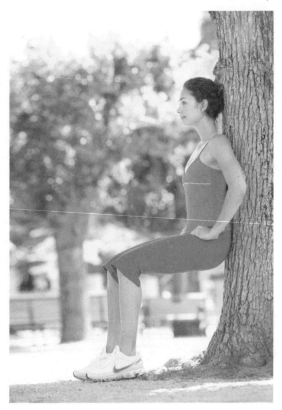

DOUBLE LIFT

TONES ABS AND BACK

Start on your hands and knees with your back flat. Tighten your abs without sucking them in. Raise and extend your left leg behind you, parallel to the ground. When you feel stable, raise and extend your right arm forward, so it's parallel to the ground. Simultaneously raise and lower your arm and leg 2 to 3 inches. Do all reps, then lower and switch sides.

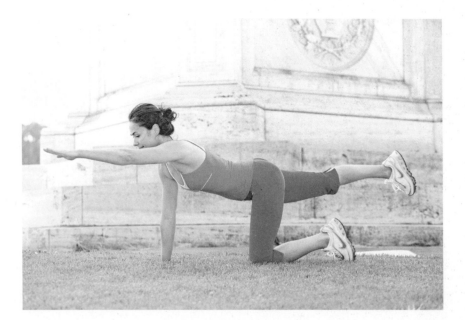

REVERSE CURL

TONES ABS

Lying faceup with your legs bent, place your hands under the small of your back and lift your feet off of the ground so your knees are over your torso. Contract your abs, pulling your knees toward your chest, and release without letting your feet touch the ground, then repeat. Avoid swinging your thighs or raising your hips; this is a very small movement.

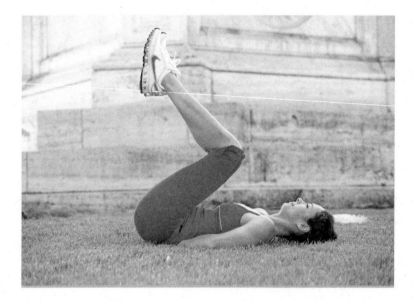

TRICEPS DIP

TONES ARMS AND BACK

Sit on the edge of a bench, wall, or railing with your hands grasping the edge and your feet flat on the ground. Walk your feet forward a few steps, with your knees over your ankles, and shift your hips just off the bench. Bend your elbows back as you lower your hips to just below bench level. Straighten your arms, pressing your body back up. (If your shoulders feel strained, don't dip as low.)

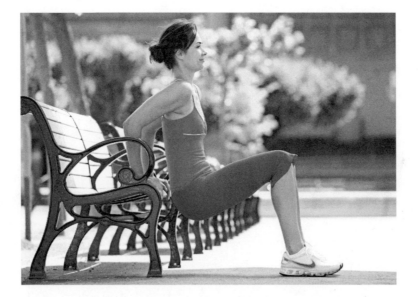

PUSHUP

TONES CHEST, ARMS, AND SHOULDERS

Get down on your hands and knees. Walk your hands forward and lower your hips until your torso forms a straight diagonal line from your shoulders to your hips to your knees. Spread your hands slightly wider than your shoulders, with your fingers pointing forward. Bend your elbows out to the sides as you lower your chest almost to the ground. Straighten your arms to push back up.

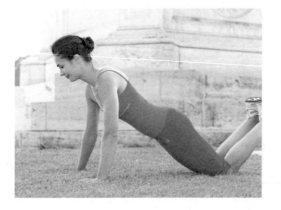 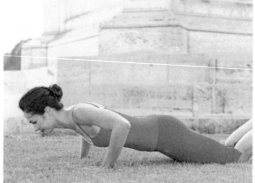

Walk 3

In 60 minutes: Burn off fat

Lose three times as much fat with high-intensity interval training. Instead of coasting along at the same speed, this routine shifts gears, alternately revving your pace to a calorie-blasting speed walk (or jumping jacks) and then slowing down so you can recover and do it again. The result: You'll maximize fat loss by burning calories at a higher rate for hours after your workout.

YOUR PLAN AT A GLANCE

TIME	PACE*	INTENSITY LEVEL**
Start	Warmup	3–4
2:00	Brisk walk	5–6
7:00	Calorie blast—speed walk or jumping jacks	8–9
9:00	Easy walk	4–5
10:00	Strong walk	6–7
15:00	Calorie blast—speed walk or jumping jacks	8–9
17:00	Easy walk	4–5
18:00	Strong walk	6–7
23:00	Calorie blast—speed walk or jumping jacks	8–9
26:00	Easy walk	4–5
27:00	Strong walk	6–7
32:00	Calorie blast—speed walk or jumping jacks	8–9
36:00	Easy walk	4–5
37:00	Strong walk	6–7
42:00	Calorie blast—speed walk or jumping jacks	8–9
47:00	Easy walk	4–5
48:00	Strong walk	6–7
53:00	Calorie blast—speed walk or jumping jacks	8–9
58:00	Cooldown	3–4
60:00	Finish	

*See "Ready, Set, Go" on page 137 for all pace descriptions.

**Based on a 1–10 scale, with 1 equivalent to sitting on the sofa and 10 equivalent to sprinting.

chapter 18

GENTLE MOVES FOR YOUR BODY AND SOUL

Build strength, lower blood pressure, and much more
with the ancient art of tai chi

Deep breathing. Slow movements. Meditation. On paper, tai chi sounds more like a spa session than a workout program, which may be why it's such a great choice for beginning-level exercisers. But this traditional Chinese discipline offers serious health benefits, including improvements in muscle tone, strength, and bone density. Tai chi has also been shown to lower blood pressure and improve heart health.

For people with diabetes, tai chi has even more to offer: One study of people with type 2 diabetes found that those who participated in a 12-week tai chi program brought down their A1c test levels (short for "glycated hemoglobin A1c"), which is a measurement of blood sugar levels over time.

Other studies indicate that regular tai chi sessions can improve balance and mobility for people who have developed peripheral neuropathy, which is nerve damage in the hands and feet. Tai chi even has been known to bolster immunity for people with type 2 diabetes. This is a good thing, because being sick can cause blood sugar levels to rise.

"This practice has been used for thousands of years to strengthen the body as it eases the mind," says David-Dorian Ross, a seven-time medalist in national and international tai chi competitions, who designed the following workout. One tai chi session takes just minutes, but its relaxing-yet-energizing effects last for hours.

Getting started: Do these postures in order, as slowly as possible, flowing from one step and posture to the next. Once you've completed all the postures, repeat the routine, working opposite arms and legs (substitute left for right and vice versa in the exercise instructions). Perform this gentle routine every day.

OPEN THE DOOR

Start by focusing on an object in front of you. Picture it as 12 o'clock on an imaginary clock. You'll use this to visualize where your body should be during the following moves. Next, stand tall, with your knees soft, your feet together, and your arms at your sides. Slowly step your left foot to the side so your feet are shoulder-width apart. Gently raise both of your arms in front of you to chest height, with your palms facing down, then slightly bend your elbows and slowly lower your arms to waist level as you bend your knees. You should sink 3 to 4 inches. (You'll face 12 o'clock for this entire exercise.)

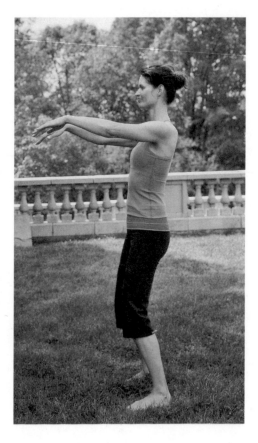 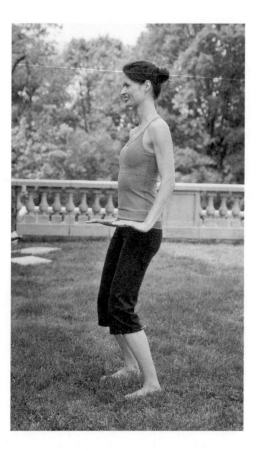

PARTING THE HORSE'S MANE

Wrap your arms around an imaginary beach ball in front of your chest, with your right hand on top, palm down, and your left hand on bottom, palm up. Turn to your left (toward 9 o'clock), and step forward with your left foot into a lunge, with your right foot still facing 12 o'clock. As you lunge, extend your left arm forward from hip to shoulder level, palm up, as you bring your right arm back and lower to waist level, with your palm down.

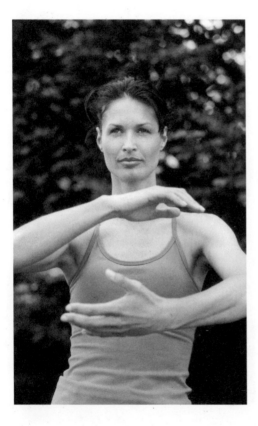
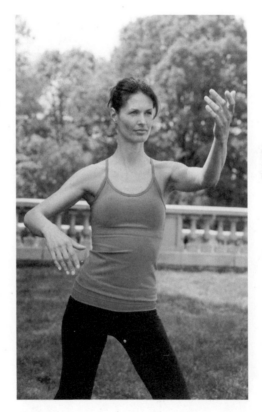

ROOSTER STANDS ON ONE LEG

With your left arm still extended and your right arm bent, straighten your left leg, keeping your knee soft. Slowly raise your right knee in front of you to waist level, dropping your left arm down to hip level, turning your palm facedown, as you simultaneously raise your right arm in front of you, with your palm cupped and facing left. Your right elbow is bent and above your right knee. You'll still be facing 9 o'clock.

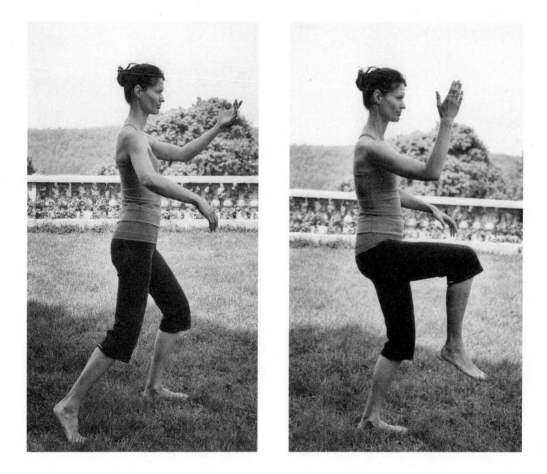

STEP UP AND KICK WITH HEEL

Put your right foot down as you cross your hands over each other in front of your chest. Shift your weight to your right foot and lift your left knee until your left thigh is parallel to the ground, raising your arms in front of you to about chest level. Open your hips and rotate your bent knee slightly out to the side. Slowly spread your arms and extend out to your sides, with your elbows slightly bent and your palms open. Slowly straighten your left leg, and press your heel forward as if you were kicking something; you'll be kicking toward 7 o'clock.

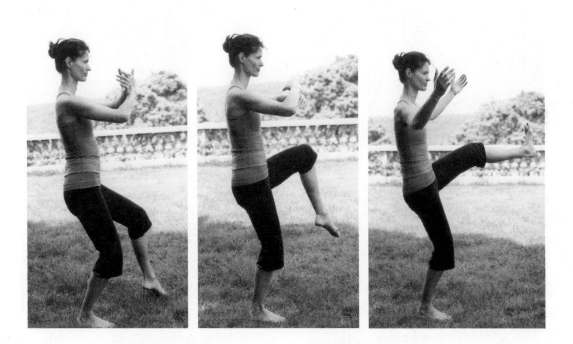

CLOSE THE DOOR

Drop your left foot and shift your weight onto it. Step your right foot back so it's pointing toward 12 o'clock and pivot your body so it also faces 12 o'clock as you circle your hands together, crossing your wrists at your waist, with your palms up. Raise them in front of your face, separate them, then let your hands float back down to your sides, with your palms down, as you straighten your legs. Bring your feet back together, and finish with a little bow.

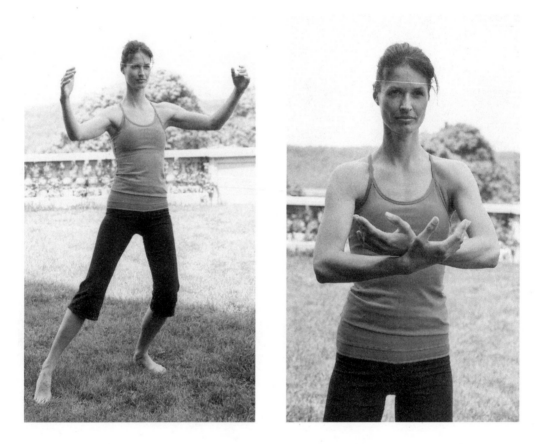

chapter 19

SLIMMING YOGA

Lose stubborn belly flab and tone up all over
with this fast, easy plan

Yoga is a known stress buster, but it's also one of the most effective workouts for fighting stubborn fat stores, especially the ones that crop up after age 40. The reason: Studies show that yoga lowers levels of stress hormones and increases insulin sensitivity—a signal to your body to burn food as fuel rather than store it as fat. The following workout will do just that while firming up your arms, legs, butt, and abs. Start now to see results in as little as 3 weeks.

Workout at a glance

What you need: A yoga mat or carpeted space

How to do it: Follow this routine at least 3 times a week, holding each move 1 time for 3 to 5 deep breaths, unless otherwise noted. Start with the main move for each exercise. If it's too difficult, do the make-it-easier variation. If it's not challenging enough, try the make-it-harder option.

For faster results: Hold each pose for 5 to 8 breaths and increase repetitions (where noted) by 2 or 3.

CRESCENT

FIRMS ABS, HIPS, AND THIGHS

Stand with your feet together, with your toes forward and your arms at your sides. Inhale and raise your arms overhead, reaching your fingertips toward the ceiling. Exhale, and bend forward from your hips, bringing your hands to the floor (it's okay to bend your knees). Inhale, and as you exhale, step your right leg back into a lunge (with your left knee bent about 90 degrees, your knee over your ankle, and your right leg extended and on the ball of your foot). Inhale and raise your arms overhead, with your gaze forward. Hold, then return to standing and repeat, stepping your left leg back.

Make it easier: Lower your right knee to touch the floor as you step back into a lunge, and rest your hands on your left thigh.

Make it harder: From the end position, inhale and arch your torso, arms, and head backward, gazing at your fingertips.

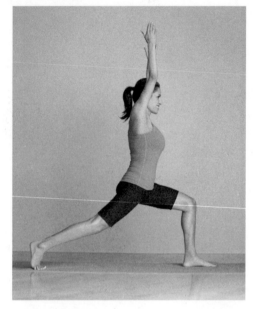

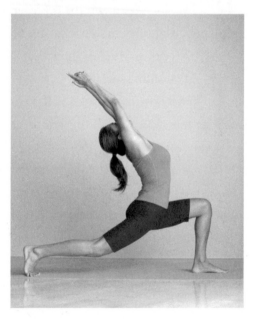

WILLOW

FIRMS SIDES OF ABS

Stand with your feet together, arms at your sides. Place the sole of your left foot on the inside of your right thigh, with your knee bent to the side. Touch your palms in front of your chest for 2 breaths. On the third inhale, extend your arms up, with your fingertips toward the ceiling. Exhale, and on the inhale, bend your torso to the left. Exhale and straighten. Repeat 3 to 5 times, pressing your foot into your thigh; switch sides.

Make it easier: Keep your left foot on your calf or touch your toes to the floor for balance.

Make it harder: Close your eyes as you balance and bend.

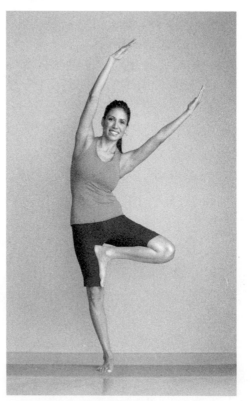

ROCKING BOAT

FIRMS ABS AND BACK

Sit with your knees bent, with your feet on the floor and your hands on your thighs. With your torso straight and your head in line with your body, lean back about 45 degrees, raising your feet so your calves are parallel to the floor and your toes are pointed. On an inhale, extend your arms and legs, keeping your legs together. Exhale, and as you inhale, lower your torso and legs 3 to 4 inches so your body forms a wider V shape. Exhale and raise your torso and legs. Repeat 3 to 5 times.

Make it easier: Hold the backs of your thighs with your hands, and keep your legs bent. Lower your torso only.

Make it harder: Once in the wider V position, extend your arms overhead.

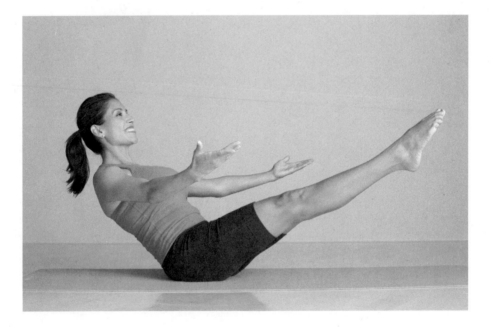

HOVER

FIRMS SHOULDERS, ARMS, ABS, AND BACK

Begin in a pushup position on your toes with arms straight, with your hands below your shoulders and your body in line from your head to your heels. On an exhale, lower your chest toward the floor, bending your elbows back, with your arms close to your body and your abs tight. Hold a few inches above the floor.

Make it easier: Begin on your hands and knees, and walk your hands forward until your body is in line from your head to your knees.

Make it harder: While holding the hover, lift your left leg 6 to 12 inches, pause, and lower. Do 3 to 5 times, then switch legs.

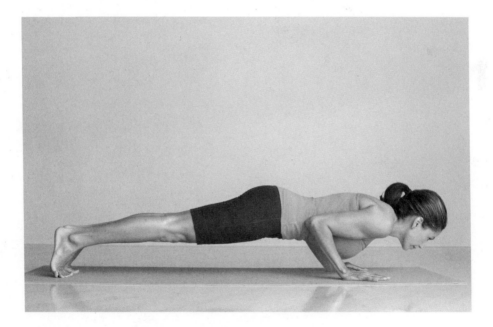

CHAIR

FIRMS BUTT AND THIGHS

Stand with your feet together, with your toes forward and your arms at your sides. Inhale and raise your arms overhead, with your palms facing each other. Exhale and sit back about 45 degrees, keeping your knees behind your toes and your abs tight to support your back; gaze forward.

Make it easier: Do the move with your feet hip-distance apart, with your hands on your thighs, and bend only about 30 degrees.

Make it harder: After you sit back, lift your heels off the floor, balancing on the balls of your feet (your knees will be in front of your toes); gaze up at your fingertips.

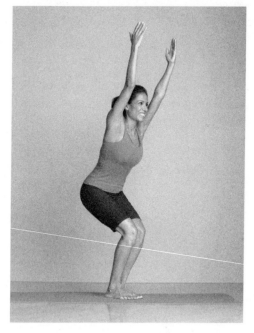

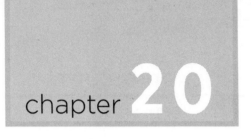

chapter 20

THE BALLERINA WORKOUT

Love your legs! Five easy, dance-inspired moves to sculpt a lean, shapely lower body

You don't have to aspire to *Dancing with the Stars* to get the slim, toned legs of a ballroom champion. To sculpt muscle fast, try this graceful—yet effective—workout created by Tina de Lemps, a former professional dancer and designer of the Ballerina Legs workout in New York City.

Workout at a Glance

What you need: A sturdy chair and a resistance band (optional).

How to do it: Follow the routine 3 times a week on nonconsecutive days. Start with 1 set of 10 repetitions of each move (unless otherwise indicated). As you become stronger, do 1 or 2 additional sets. Try the main move first. If it's too tough, start with the make-it-easier option. For an added challenge, do the make-it-harder variation.

For quicker results: Add cardio spurts: March in place or do jumping jacks.

CARDIO CURTSY

Stand with your feet hip-width apart, with your toes point-ing out. Hold a chair with your left hand (like a dancer at a barre), with your right arm at your side. Cross your right leg behind you, bending both of your knees as if you were curtsying. At the same time, sweep your right arm up and over, bending gently toward your left. Straighten your legs and lift your right knee to the side, bending your torso to bring your right elbow toward your right knee. Without pausing, repeat 25 times as quickly as you can while main-taining good form. Switch sides.

Make it easier: Don't lift your knee toward your elbow. Instead, keep your right toes on the floor as you slide your foot out to the right, and bring your right elbow to the side.

Make it harder: As you lift your knee toward your elbow, rise up onto the ball of your left foot.

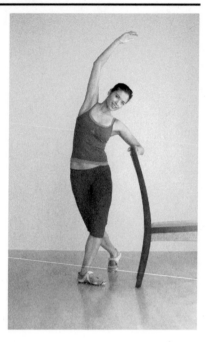

BIG KICKS

Stand with your heels together, with your toes turned out, your left hand holding a chair, and your right arm over your head. Keeping your abs tight, raise your right leg forward as high as you can without arching your back. (It may be only several inches.) As you lower your right arm to the side, circle your right leg out to the side without lowering it. Continue, circling your leg behind you as you tip your torso forward, extending your right arm in front of you. Lower your right foot to the floor, returning to the starting position. Do all repetitions, then switch sides.

Make it easier: Break the move into 3 parts: Raise your leg forward, then lower to the starting position; repeat to the side and then to the back.

Make it harder: To provide resistance as you kick, tie an exercise band around your right ankle, and step on the loose end with your left foot. The shorter the band is between your left foot and right ankle, the harder it will be. Hold each kick for 3 counts.

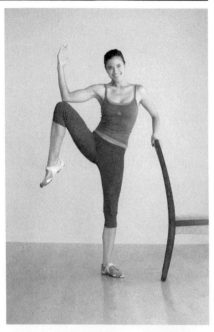

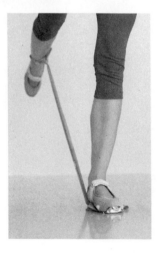

SCISSOR LEGS

Lie on your left side with your left arm under your head, with your right hand on the floor and your legs in line with your torso. Lift your right leg about 2 feet and hold while you lift your left leg about 1 foot. Pause, then lower your left leg, followed by your right leg. Do all repetitions, then switch sides.

Make it easier: Bend at your hips so your legs are slightly in front of your body. Lift and lower the top leg only.

Make it harder: Squeezing your legs together, lift them about 1 foot off the floor. Pause, then raise your top leg about 1 foot higher, still holding your lower leg off the floor. Lower your top leg back to your bottom leg, then slowly lower both legs.

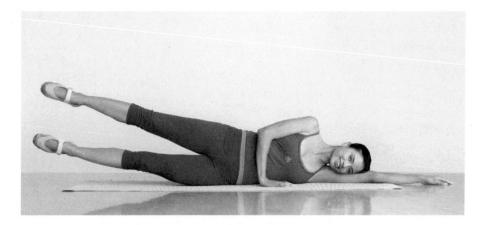

FUNKY BALLERINA

Stand with your heels facing each other, with your toes out, your right hand holding a chair, and your left hand on your hip. Plié, bending your knees to about 45 degrees. Lift your heels off the floor and squeeze your butt, tilting your pelvis forward and back 1 time. Lower your heels and straighten your legs for 1 repetition.

Make it easier: Lie faceup with your heels together and your knees pointing out so your legs form a diamond. Lift your butt off the floor and hold as you tilt your pelvis up and down once, then lower to the floor for 1 repetition.

Make it harder: Hold the plié position with your knees bent to 45 degrees and your heels lifted as you tilt your pelvis back and forth for all repetitions.

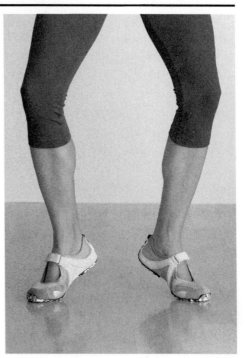

SLIDE AND REACH

Stand with your heels together, with your toes turned out, your left hand holding a chair, and your right arm out to the side. Slide your right foot about 3 feet to the right, and bend your knees to lower into a deep plié squat while reaching your right arm overhead and bending toward your left side. Stand back up, sliding your right foot to the starting position. Rise up onto the balls of your feet, then immediately lower. Do all repetitions, then switch sides.

Make it easier: Place the chair in front of you, holding it with both hands (don't reach or bend to the side).

Make it harder: Tie the ends of an exercise band in a knot, and loop it around your calves. Perform the move with this added resistance.

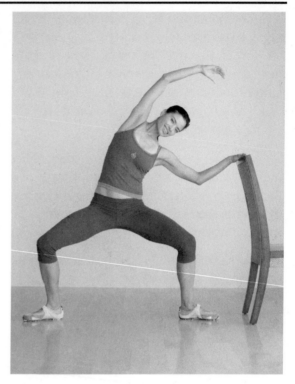

chapter 21

THE HAVE-IT-YOUR-WAY WORKOUT PLAN

Choose a workout to meet your shape-up goals. Getting started (or jumping back in) has never been easier!

Not exercising as often as you'd like? We all get sidetracked now and then. So we asked top fitness experts to create three routines that anyone can ease into—all take 20 minutes or less. In a study from Pennington Biomedical Research Center in Baton Rouge, Louisiana, exercising 15 minutes a day three or four times a week was all that women needed for shedding abdominal fat. Try one plan—or all three! In just 2 weeks, you'll notice a tighter belly, a loss of 1 to 2 pounds, better muscle tone (and higher metabolism), and more energy!

BOOST METABOLISM WITH A STRENGTH CIRCUIT

"I gain weight more easily since turning 40."

This full-body circuit routine—doing one strength exercise after another without rest—builds fat-burning muscle fast while targeting belly bulge with ab moves. A University of

Your Workout at a Glance

Weeks 1 and 2: Perform the routine 3 times a week on nonconsecutive days. Using light dumbbells (3 to 5 pounds), do 1 set of 12 to 15 repetitions of each move in the order given. Do the exercises without stopping—or rest for no longer than 15 seconds.

Weeks 3 and 4: Repeat the circuit twice so you're doing a total of 2 sets per exercise.

Keep it up: After 4 weeks, try increasing the weights by 1 to 3 pounds. You'll burn fat, tone muscle, and build bone even faster!

Hawaii study found that circuit-training raises your heart rate higher than vigorous running (15 beats per minute faster). The moves alternate between upper and lower body, so your heart works harder pumping blood up and down your body. "All that extra work means a bigger calorie burn," says Juan Carlos Santana, director of the Institute of Human Performance in Boca Raton, Florida, who designed this circuit-training workout.

LATERAL LIFT

TONES LEGS AND BUTT

Stand with your feet shoulder-width apart, with your hands on your hips, then slowly squat until your thighs are almost parallel to the ground. As you push back up, lift your left leg out to the side as if you were going to step out. Your leg should create a 45-degree angle with the ground. Hold for 1 second, then return your foot to the ground. Squat with both of your feet once more, then repeat with your right leg. That's 1 repetition.

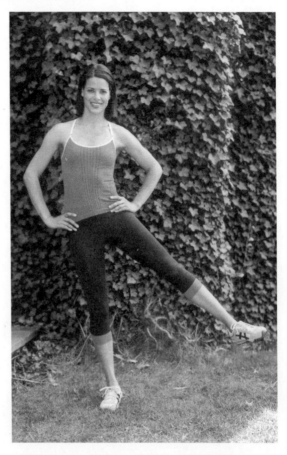

CHEST FLY AND PRESS

TONES SHOULDERS, CHEST, AND TRICEPS

Lie faceup with a dumbbell in each hand, with your elbows and knees bent and your feet flat. Raise your arms above your chest, with your palms facing each other. Slowly lower your arms out to the sides as far as you can, then raise back to the starting position. Next, bend your arms and lower the weights until your upper arms touch the ground, with your elbows out to the sides to form a T. Straighten your arms, pressing the weights above you. That's 1 repetition.

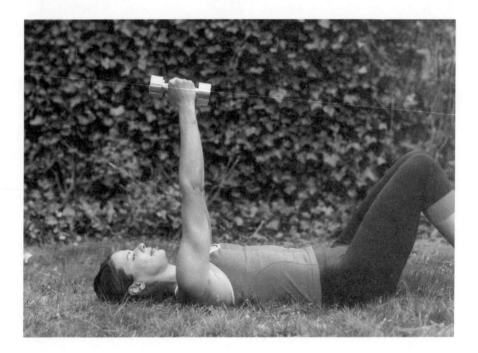

PLIÉ SQUAT

TONES LEGS AND BUTT

Stand straight with your feet wider than shoulder-width apart, with your toes pointed out. Hold one end of a dumbbell in each hand in front of you, with your arms hanging straight down. Squat slowly until your thighs are almost parallel to the ground. Slowly rise back up, pushing down on your heels to help contract your glutes and hamstrings.

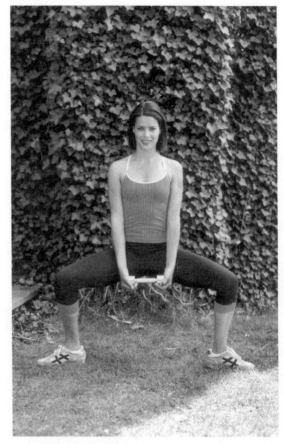

ONE-ARM ROTATION ROW

TONES BACK AND BICEPS

Stand with your right side next to a bench or bed, holding a dumbbell in your left hand. Rest your right hand and knee on the bench, and bend at your waist. Your back should be almost parallel to the ground, with your left arm hanging down and your palm facing forward. Slowly pull the weight up to your side, rotating it as you go so your palm faces behind you at the top. Lower the weight, rotating it so your palm faces forward at the bottom. Complete repetitions, then switch sides to work your right arm.

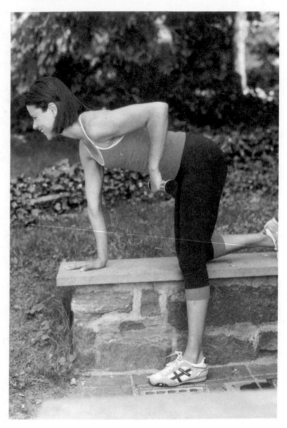

LUNGE

SHAPES LEGS AND BUTT

Stand tall with a dumbbell in each hand, with your feet hip-width apart, your arms hanging straight down at your sides, and your palms facing in. Step 2 to 3 feet forward with your left foot, and lower your body until your left thigh is almost parallel to the ground. Your right leg should be extended behind you with only the ball of your right foot on the ground. Push off from your left foot to return to the starting position, then repeat with your right leg. That's 1 repetition.

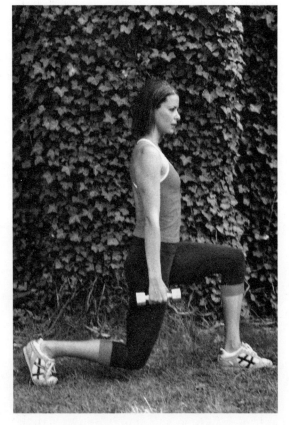

TUCK AND CRUNCH

TONES ABS

Lie faceup with your knees bent, with your feet on the ground. Touch your hands lightly to the sides of your head, pointing your elbows toward your knees. Curl your head and shoulders up as you raise your knees toward your elbows—try to touch your thighs with your elbows—then slowly lower. Avoid pulling your head forward with your hands.

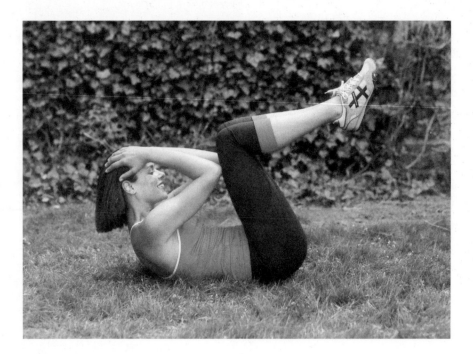

UPPERCUT

TONES SHOULDERS AND ARMS

Stand tall with a dumbbell in each hand, with your arms at your sides and your palms facing forward. Curl both weights up to your shoulders, then draw your hands in toward each other until the weights touch in front of your chest. Press the weight in your right hand above your head, with your palm facing you. Lower back to your chest, then repeat the move with your left hand. Lower back to your chest. Separate the weights so your hands are in front of your shoulders, then curl the weights back down.

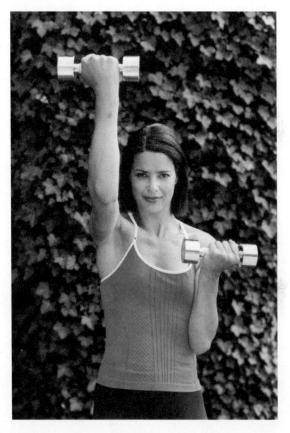

ROTATING KNEE

TONES ABS AND OBLIQUES

Lie faceup with your knees bent, with your feet on the ground and your arms out to the sides, palms facing up. Keeping your legs together, lift your butt and feet an inch off the ground, and slowly rotate your legs to the right, lowering them to the ground without touching. Hold, return to center, then twist to the left. Alternate from right to left. If the move is too intense, rest your butt on the ground between repetitions.

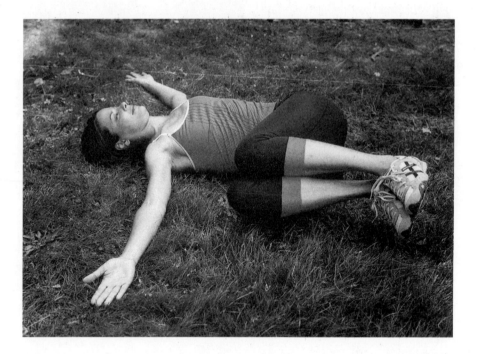

BLAST FAT BY TREADING WATER

"My joints ache."

"When you're neck-deep in water, your body weighs 10 percent of what it does on land," says Nicholas DiNubile, MD, orthopedic consultant for the Pennsylvania Ballet and author of *FrameWork: Your 7-Step Program for Healthy Muscles, Bones, and Joints*, who designed the walking and water workouts. "That helps reduce stress on joints." A recent Australian study found that subjects who used hydrotherapy had less pain, improved physical performance, and also exercised more often.

Not a swimmer? With these unique treading drills, you'll boost metabolism (burning 12½ calories per minute) and sculpt muscle without breaking out of a dog paddle.

Start Basic Tread: In water deep enough that your feet don't touch the bottom, hold your arms out at your sides underwater and trace imaginary 8s with your fingertips. Kick as necessary.

0:15 Upper-Body Tread: Keep treading water using just arms (legs crossed).

0:30 Wall Flutters: Grab the edge of the pool (hands about shoulder-width apart), and straighten your arms so that your body floats on top of the water. Kick vigorously.

0:45 Belly-Down Treat: Still floating on your belly, keep your head above the water with

Your Workout at a Glance

Do the routine 3 or 4 times weekly. You'll start by repeating our short routine 5 or 6 times (to burn 125 to 150 calories in 12 minutes), building up to 20 minutes by week 4 (250 calories). Count or watch a clock while doing each move.

Week 1: Repeat the cycle 5 or 6 times.

Week 2: Repeat the cycle 6 or 7 times.

Week 3: Repeat the cycle 7 to 9 times.

Week 4: Repeat the cycle 9 or 10 times.

Keep it up: Treading is great, but swimming can boost the calorie burn even higher. Find an instructor near you at www.clubswim.com.

your arms out. Angle your hands down, cupping them, then tread, moving only your lower arms and hands back and forth. Kick as necessary.

1:00 Belly-Up Tread: Flip onto your back, keeping your hands by your waist, just below the water. Bending your hands at the wrists, draw tiny circles with cupped hands to stay afloat. Kick as necessary.

1:15 Wall Pull-Ups: Grab the edge of the pool with both hands, and slowly push yourself up out of the water until your arms are straight, with your elbows unlocked, then lower yourself back into the water, repeating as often as you can in 15 seconds. Avoid using your feet by keeping your legs crossed throughout the move.

1:30 Rest for 30 seconds.

2:00 Repeat the cycle.

BURN MEGA CALORIES WITH WALKING

"I need to shape up fast."

Add high- and low-intensity intervals to your daily walk to make it a super fat-blaster. A University of New South Wales study found that people who exercised for 20 minutes, alternating between a high intensity for 8 seconds and a low intensity for 12 seconds, lost three times more fat than those who worked out at a constant pace for 40 minutes. In other words, intervals delivered more fat loss in half the time. This routine is a modified version of that program.

Your Workout at a Glance

Weeks 1 and 2: Three or four times a week, do either the Indoor Interval or the Outdoor Interval for a total of 20 minutes. Each routine burns about 150 calories.

Weeks 3 and 4: Walk 7 days a week. Continue your Interval workouts; on alternate days, do a 30- to 45-minute walk at a moderate speed.

Keep it up: To continue losing weight, challenge yourself: Speed up the pace of your fast intervals, raise your treadmill incline higher, or add another 10 minutes to your workouts.

How Fast Should I Go?

Warmup/Cooldown: Easy enough that you can sing

Moderate: Comfortable enough that you can talk freely

Power Walk: Brisk enough that you can talk but you'd rather not

Indoor Interval

Start: Warm up, walk at a 3- to 3.5-mph pace, and set the treadmill at a 2-degree incline.

2:00: Look at your watch, and change the incline by the second hand:

Every time your watch hits :00, raise the incline 4 to 7 degrees.

Every time your watch hits :20, lower it to 2 degrees.

18:00: Cool down, easy pace, at a 1-degree incline.

20:00: Finish

Outdoor Interval

Start: Warm up, walk at an easy pace.

2:00: Look at your watch, and change your pace by the second hand:

Every time your watch hits :00, power walk with your arms bent.

Every time your watch hits :20, walk at a moderate pace.

18:00: Cool down, walk at an easy pace.

20:00: Finish

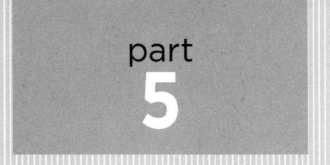

part
5

STRESS LESS

medical
BREAKTHROUGHS

R educing stress is important for your overall health, as well as for your life with diabetes. In a recent study, researchers in the Boston area found that the most stressful part of diabetes is injecting insulin. The second greatest cause of emotional distress is oral drug therapy, followed by adopting a more healthy diet. Here's the latest research on diabetes distress.

DEAL WITH DEPRESSION

Diabetes and depression have more in common than the letter D. People with diabetes commonly suffer from depression. However, researchers were curious to know if depression is as prevalent in people who are at risk for developing diabetes, and if so, what the implications of that would be.

Researchers reviewed findings from the Study to Help Improve Early evaluation and management of risk factors Leading to Diabetes (SHIELD), which included 3,530 people with type 2 diabetes, 5,051 people at high risk for developing diabetes, and 5,335 people at low risk for diabetes. The researchers asked the volunteers to fill out questionnaires assessing their quality of life and symptoms of depression.

The researchers discovered that quality of life was lower and that depression was more common for people with diabetes and those at high risk for developing it, compared with the people at low risk for developing diabetes.

"Based on these findings, people with diabetes should openly dialog with their doctors to discuss treatment for the factors causing their depression and poor quality of life so they can receive the help needed to manage all aspects of their diabetes," says Susan Grandy, PhD, study coauthor. "Additionally, individuals at high risk for diabetes but who do not have the diagnosis yet should speak with their doctor about modifying their risk factors for diabetes, such as weight, waist size, blood pressure, and cholesterol, so that they may lower their risk for developing diabetes, depression, and poor quality of life."

CHILL OUT

Flipping the bird to drivers who cut you off could increase your chances of getting diabetes. Doctors at the Cleveland Clinic measured the stress and hostility levels of 643 people and compared those figures with their insulin and glucose levels. It was found that people with high hostility levels, especially cynics, are less able to use glucose properly for energy when under stress, increasing their risk of developing diabetes.

CHECK YOUR SLEEP NUMBER

Sleeping Beauty might need a kiss from her true love to wake her, but after that, she might need a diabetologist. Researchers in Finland recently discovered that sleeping too little, and too much, are both associated with diabetes, in middle-aged women anyway.

The researchers studied almost 3,000 people, all of whom received a glucose test and answered a sleep questionnaire. The researchers found that women who slept less than 6 hours or more than 8 hours were more likely to develop diabetes. There was no such increase in the men studied.

DON'T WORRY; LIVE LONGER

Your personality may dictate when you'll die. After studying 1,633 people for 30 years, Purdue scientists found that worrying takes 16 years off your life. Negative thinking triggers the release of cortisol, a stress hormone that can be dangerous when elevated for long periods of time, says study author Dan Mroczek, PhD. Unhealthy coping techniques, such as overeating, may also contribute.

The good news is that people in the study who found a way to reduce their worry lived longer. One strategy to eliminate anxiety is to become a volunteer. Altruistic actions distract you from stress, says a study in *Psychosomatic Medicine*.

TRY SOME FLOWER POWER

Marijuana isn't Mother Nature's only herbal tranquilizer. New research from the University of Miami shows that a combination of flower extracts may be a safe and effective stress buster. Scientists discovered that anxious college students who swallowed 20 drops of a liquid containing extracts of rock rose, impatiens, clematis, star of Bethlehem, and cherry plum were significantly less stressed after 90 minutes and experienced no side effects. (One theory is that this botanical brew increases the body's production of calming endorphins.) The supplement is sold under the name Rescue Remedy ($9, www.gnc.com), but talk to your doctor before taking any herbal aid.

BLOW OFF STRESS!

Call it thumb sucking for grown-ups: To calm down fast, put the tip of your thumb in your mouth, make a seal, blow while puffing out your cheeks, and hold for 5 to 10 seconds. The increased pressure in your chest cavity stimulates the vagus nerve—a cord that runs from the brain to the abdomen—limiting blood flow to the heart. The instant result: a slower heartbeat.

"We ask people to do this before we give them medication," says Ben Abo, an emergency medicine specialist in Pittsburgh. "And it works just as well for everyday jitters."

BET ON HAPPINESS

Winning isn't everything: Just buying a lottery ticket gives you an emotional payoff. Neuroscientists have found that the mere anticipation and excitement of a possible windfall lights up the same circuits in the brain as winning does. Our suggestion: Save your dollar and enter a free sweepstakes or giveaway instead. We're betting you'll reap the same rewards—without spending a cent!

SOOTHE YOUR JANGLED NERVES

Popping pistachios may limit the toll that stress takes on you. Penn State nutritionists found that having a handful (1½ ounces) daily for 1 month helped keep study subjects' blood pressure down in a stressful situation. With 3 ounces came an extra bonus: increased artery relaxation, which may lighten your heart's workload. A 1½-ounce serving has 240 calories and 10 grams of fat.

HAVE A KISS

Here's a new meaning for the term "chocolate lover." Doctors at the Mind Lab in England asked six couples to savor squares of dark chocolate and then smooch, all while hooked up to brain and heart monitors. Both tasks made neurological sparks fly and hearts flutter, but chocolate doubled excitation rates in the brain's pleasure center, especially in women. Cocoa's blend of fat, sugar, and caffeine lasts longer than a kiss, say researchers. For the best buzz, let a small piece dissolve slowly.

SLEEP ON IT

Here's proof that a good snooze makes you smarter. Volunteers presented with a brain teaser were far more likely to solve it after a full night's rest than those asked to figure it out right away or even several hours later, report Harvard researchers.

"Sometimes, memorizing the facts isn't enough," says study leader Matthew Walker,

PhD, an assistant professor of psychology at Harvard Medical School. "Sleep can knit ideas together: You go to bed with pieces of the puzzle and awaken with the picture complete."

PLAY DIRTY, BE HAPPY

Digging in the dirt may boost your mood and help you cope with stress, says a study from the University of Bristol in the United Kingdom. Researchers found that mice that inhaled bacteria commonly found in soil tried harder to work out a stressful problem (escaping from a pool of water); mice that didn't sniff the bacteria gave up more easily. The soil-loving bugs are thought to stimulate the release of mood-enhancing chemicals in the brain. So take a big whiff of that compost pile. Then plant some bulbs for next spring.

The percentage of busy women who say sleep is the first thing they sacrifice, according to the National Sleep Foundation: 52 percent

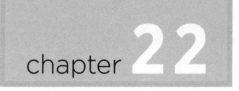

chapter 22

THE BEST ZEN FOR YOU

Take on a new level of calm with these fresh twists
on tried-and-true de-stressors

Want to find the ultimate in peace and happiness? The key is to make sure you haven't fallen into a relaxation rut. If your usual stress buster isn't soothing your anxiety like it used to, you need to try something new to boost peace of mind. We found five cool variations on popular pastimes that can settle your nerves in record time.

IF YOU WIND DOWN WITH A BATH, TRY A NATURAL HOT SPRING

Move over, Mr. Bubble. It's worth going the extra tension-taming mile to plunge into a natural spring.

"Soaking in hot springs lowers levels of the stress hormone cortisol, which reduces inflammation and built-up strain in your ligaments and joints," says Pamela Peeke, MD, MPH, an assistant professor of medicine at the University of Maryland School of Medicine.

Some top spots include Dunton Hot Springs in Colorado ($75 for the day, including lunch), the Hot Springs Resort & Spa in North Carolina (from $12), and Ojo Caliente Mineral Springs in New Mexico (from $16). For more ideas, visit www.trails.com, which has a substantial database of hot springs, including secluded ones that require a hike through the woods.

IF YOU EMPTY YOUR MIND WITH MEDITATION, TRY QIGONG

Shake up your seated practice with qigong (pronounced chee-gong, which means "energy work"), an active Chinese meditation routine that mixes and matches hundreds of fluid, graceful dancelike exercises. By focusing on these repetitive movements and your breathing, your mind pushes aside intrusive thoughts and elicits the body's relaxation response: Your heart rate slows down, and blood pressure, adrenaline, and cortisol levels drop.

Classes are often held at YMCAs, gyms, and community or wellness centers and cost around $10 to $20 per session. To find a local instructor, go to the National Qigong Association's Web site, www.nqa.org.

IF YOU WALK OFF A BAD DAY, TRY A LABYRINTH STROLL

These mazelike paths, which date back thousands of years, have grown in popularity, thanks in part to promising research documenting meditation's effects on blood pressure, cortisol levels, and other markers of stress reduction, according to M. Kay Sandor, PhD, an associate professor of nursing at the University of Texas Medical Branch at Galveston. Labyrinths can be inlaid on church floors, marked by stones in a garden, mowed into grassy fields, or painted on the ground in public parks. Walkers follow a single circuitous route free of wrong turns or dead ends toward the center. Most courses take about 20 minutes to complete, but Dr. Sandor suggests that you go at your own pace. When you reach the center, take as much time as you'd like for reflection—then retrace your steps back out.

Finding a labyrinth is relatively easy: More than 1,000 hospitals, spas, schools, churches, and wellness centers in the United States have installed labyrinths on-site. (You can also search www.veriditas.net to find one near you.)

IF YOU REFRESH YOUR SPIRITS BY HIKING, TRY GEOCACHING

A high-tech version of an old-fashioned scavenger hunt, geocaching has become an increasingly popular weekend activity since global positioning system (GPS) signals were made accessible to the public in 2000. Participants log on to a free geocaching Web site to get the coordinates of "caches"—secret stashes of everyday objects hidden across the world. Any person, team, or organization can set up and monitor a cache according to safe geocaching rules. In fact, there are already more than 600,000 caches scattered around the globe. Each cache is ranked according to the difficulty of the hunt and the terrain, so you can choose a trek that matches your fitness level. Players plug the specific coordinates into a handheld GPS device that guides them as they walk through woods, snowshoe along trails, or hike through mountain meadows.

When you find a cache, you can take the trinket out of it and leave a new treasure behind for the next person to discover. Most caches also include a logbook for you to sign and date with a brief description of your journey. Check out www.geocaching.com to find cache coordinates in your area.

IF YOU DECOMPRESS WITH MASSAGE, TRY REIKI

Japanese for "universal life energy," this bodywork method involves gentle touch or none at all. Reiki therapists believe that they can channel energy through their hands and transmit it to the patient, promoting balance and healing. During a Reiki session, which typically lasts between 60 and 90 minutes, you'll lie on a massage table, fully dressed, while the therapist places her hands in various positions around your head, torso, legs, and feet. Studies have shown that Reiki reduces anxiety and blood pressure.

To find a local Reiki therapist, contact the International Association of Reiki Professionals (www.iarp.org) or the International Center for Reiki Training (www.reiki.org).

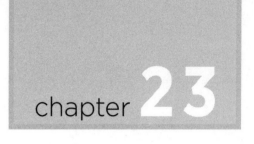

chapter 23

THE POWER
OF PLUCK

Develop resilience and come through tough times
happier and healthier

ngela Madsen was a military police officer in the US Marine Corps when
she injured her back so severely that she had to take an early discharge. She
needed surgery, and when she awoke from anesthesia, she learned that her
spinal column had been pierced and that she was partially paralyzed from
the waist down. She was told that she wouldn't walk again for a year or two, and maybe
never. "I did exactly what many people do after something like that. I went through a
period of feeling hopeless," says the 47-year-old single mother and grandmother from Long
Beach, California.

And at first, her situation did seem hopeless. She lost her job as a mechanical engineer.
She began to gain weight, ballooning to more than 300 pounds. Then came a turning
point. A remark by a doctor, who called her physical condition "a waste of a human life,"
flipped a switch. She vowed she would do whatever it took to get her life back. Today, 14
years later, Madsen is training to be the first woman with a disability to row across the

Atlantic. It will cap more than a decade of awards for rowing, swimming, surfing, basketball, shot put, javelin, weight lifting, and even billiards.

Madsen is what researchers call *resilient*—someone who is able to rebound from whatever difficulty life brings. She is one of those people who make us wonder how we would fare if our own mettle were tested. Would we bounce back or be crushed by the pressure?

"From birth, some people do have a greater capacity to be resilient in the face of adversity," says Robert Brooks, PhD, an assistant clinical professor of psychology at Harvard Medical School and coauthor of *The Power of Resilience*. "But biology is not destiny. That's where life experience comes in." Indeed, a growing body of research on those who've survived some of life's toughest trials—rape, a life-threatening illness, a child's death—reveals a handful of traits that resilient people share and other people can develop.

THEY TAKE CONTROL OF THEIR LIVES

As part of her recovery, Madsen returned to the one thing that empowered her in the past: sports. She got involved in a women's wheelchair basketball league, and she taught herself to surf on her knees.

Experts say she tapped into one of the most important traits resilient people share: They don't see themselves as victims whose fate is in the hands of others. "It's easy to blame other people for your problems and wait until they fix them," says psychiatrist Steven Wolin, MD, coauthor with Sybil Wolin, PhD, of *The Resilient Self: How Survivors of Troubled Families Rise Above Adversity*. "But then you never get to rise to the occasion and witness your own strength. If you think of yourself as a problem solver, life goes very differently."

In a 12-year study tracing one of the subsidiaries of AT&T, Illinois Bell Telephone Company researchers found that employees who thrived during the notorious upheaval had three characteristics in common: They saw problems as challenges, were committed to facing them head-on, and looked to influence their own outcomes. Although Bell experienced massive layoffs (nearly half of its 26,000 employees) and most of the remaining workforce was traumatized, the resilient employees had fewer stress-related illnesses than those who felt helpless.

What you can do: Identify your strengths. Recall those moments when you triumphed over adversity, and give yourself credit. Resilient people learn from hard times, and they also acknowledge their own fortitude. In Dr. Wolin's work with children and adults who grew up in dysfunctional families, he found that those who did better in life have "survivor's pride."

"Resilient people focus on what they can influence and don't spend time on things they can't," says Dr. Brooks. "Once you develop that sense of personal control, you begin to realize that you are the author of your own life."

THEY FORGE CONNECTIONS

As a child, Ned Hallowell, MD, faced some tough odds. "I had a bipolar father, an alcoholic and abusive stepfather, an alcoholic mother, and two learning disabilities—ADD and dyslexia," he says. Although his father was a gifted teacher and his mother was devoted to her son, their troubles deeply affected him. "People with that profile often end up in jail or a mental hospital, at best eking out a marginal existence."

When Dr. Hallowell was 10, his mother sent him to boarding school. "I didn't have a sign around my neck that said 'troubled child, help me.' But I attached myself to several teachers who took me under their wing," he explains. "They saved my life." Today, he's a prominent psychiatrist, a happily married father of three, and the author of a dozen books, several on the value of what he calls "human moments"—our meaningful connections to other people.

Studies of people who don't have a strong family support system find that the most resilient, like Dr. Hallowell, seek aid from others. "In research on abused children, those who were resilient as adults had at least one person who stood by them," says Dr. Brooks. Some researchers speculate that developing connections to others may be our most important emotional survival skill. Studies have shown that people who had many relationships—with family, friends, neighbors, and coworkers, and even within church and community groups—actually lived longer than those who had the fewest.

What you can do: Make time for what matters. A 2006 Duke University study reported that the number of Americans who say they have no one to talk to about important subjects has nearly tripled since 1985. "You need to find time for what you value—

family and friends, your pet, your garden, spirituality," says Dr. Hallowell. "People and hobbies will sustain you in the long run."

THEY ALLOW PAIN TO SPUR GROWTH

In 1983, at the peak of her career as a nature photographer, Linda Joy Montgomery learned she was going blind, the result of nerve damage caused by type 1 diabetes. She was terrified. "Photography wasn't just a job, it was my mission," says Montgomery, 54, of Black Mountain, North Carolina. "I didn't know how I was going to function." But as she listened to her doctor's crushing diagnosis, she heard a voice from the inside. "It said, 'This is not the end, this is the beginning,' " she recalls. "Although I still had doubts and fears, I believed this was happening for a reason."

Although Montgomery could no longer express herself through her camera and photographs, she began writing poetry. In 1989, she published a book called *Silent Strength* that combined her nature photographs with her inspirational verse. She also found a new calling as a motivational speaker and created the True Vision Institute, teaching elementary students how to tap into their intuition and imagination.

Montgomery's ability to grow and find meaning in her misfortune is no aberration. Studies of victims of rape and incest, life-threatening illness, natural disasters, and combat, as well as Holocaust survivors and parents of chronically ill children, show that resilient people find the proverbial silver lining by reinventing themselves. Some gain a new appreciation for life; others, a renewed closeness to the people they love. "After overcoming a challenge, you develop a deep self-confidence and sense of optimism: 'I've been here, done that, and I'll survive,'" says Al Siebert, PhD, author of *The Resiliency Advantage*, who has interviewed hundreds of such survivors.

What you can do: Accentuate the positive. Cultivate your childlike curiosity; grab every opportunity to laugh, spend time with friends. When trouble strikes, these will be your best resources. University of North Carolina at Chapel Hill researcher Barbara Fredrickson, PhD, and others have found that during bad times, feeling positive—making plans for the future, expressing love and gratitude—helps people bounce back more quickly. "You need to find ways to adjust to fluctuating circumstances," says Dr. Siebert.

THEY INSIST ON CHANGING THE WORLD

Ken Druck, PhD, an organizational psychologist and high-profile executive coach in San Diego, has taught resilience skills to top execs at companies such as Microsoft, IBM, and Pfizer. But in 1996, Druck experienced every parent's worst nightmare: His 21-year-old daughter, Jenna, was killed in a bus accident while studying abroad in India. That's when he learned that all the resilience in the world couldn't prepare him for the death of a child.

"After my daughter died, I wanted to die," says Druck. "While at no point was I suicidal, I, like many bereaved parents, had lost my sense of purpose. All the goodness had gone from my life."

Yet before the year was out, Druck, still reeling, had set the wheels in motion for his new life. To honor his daughter, who was San Diego's Young Woman Entrepreneur at age 9, he established the Jenna Druck Foundation. Its Young Women's Leadership Program provides leadership training for thousands of girls each year. A second program, Families Helping Families, offers free support services to bereaved families, individuals, and communities after the death of a child. Druck and his staff were on the scene following the Columbine High School shootings, at Ground Zero after the September 11 attacks, and in New Orleans after Hurricane Katrina.

"It helped me heal," says Druck. "When you lose someone, love endures. But it hurts to not be able to express that love in the way that we're all accustomed to. Starting a foundation and doing good things every day in my daughter's name was another way for me to say 'I love you.'"

What you can do: Always give before you take: Helping others may be part of a human self-righting mechanism. In a study of rescue workers who dug through the rubble after the Oklahoma City bombing, most, although understandably distressed, had few or no symptoms of post-traumatic stress disorder afterward. More than one-third told researchers that even though their job involved the removal of human remains, it still gave them a sense of "relief and closure." "I once heard that in German concentration camps, there were a few men who always gave away their last morsel of food to other people," says Brooks. "That illustrates that you have the freedom to choose your attitude in any given set of circumstances, to control the only thing you can control in life—you."

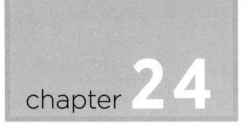

chapter 24

THE HAPPINESS FACTOR

Tap into your bright side

J oie de vivre. We all know people whose engagement with life can only be described as joyful. Fittingly, nature rewards these happy-go-lucky types: Being optimistic in middle age increases life span by at least 7.5 years—even after accounting for age, gender, socioeconomic status, and physical health, according to a large Yale University survey. What's behind their hardiness: They minimize the destructive effects of stress. "Of course, optimists get stressed," says David Snowdon, MPH, PhD, a professor of neurology at the University of Kentucky who studies aging. "But they automatically turn the response off much more quickly and return to a positive mental and physical state." Longevity experts say four habits are at the heart of a sunny disposition.

THEY WORK THEIR CELL PHONES

Perhaps your neighborhood gossip is on to something: All that chitchat keeps her plugged in to a thriving social network, and people who socialize at least once a week

The Best Kind of Pessimist

If you're an irritable sort who thinks of your eternally cheery neighbor as a delusional Polly-anna, are you doomed to poor health? Not if you're an active pessimist, a feisty spirit who loves to complain, criticize, and generally mix it up with others—but then takes action. "Active pessimists do battle with life. Being that engaged is actually good for them and can provide some of the same benefits that optimists enjoy," says Toni Antonucci, PhD, director of the Life Course Development Program of the Institute for Social Research at the University of Michigan. Passive pessimists, on the other hand, feel paralyzed by gloom, have given up on themselves and life, and will likely live fewer years because of their bummer attitude.

are more likely to live longer, keep their brains sharp, and prevent heart attacks.

One reason: "Just talking on the phone to a friend has the immediate effect of lowering your blood pressure and cortisol levels," says Teresa Seeman, PhD, a professor of medicine and epidemiology at UCLA. "Our research shows that having good long-term relation-ships provides as many physical benefits as being active or a nonsmoker."

Make the effort to connect with the friends you already have. Call now, and before you hang up, schedule a lunch date. Personal contact is even better.

THEY EXPRESS GRATITUDE

Buoy your spirits by recording happy events on paper, your computer, or a PDA. People who write about all the things they are thankful for are optimistic about the upcoming week and more satisfied overall with their lives, according to a University of California, Davis, study. They also feel physically stronger. "It's hard to be bitter and mad when you're feeling grateful," says Sonja Lyubomirsky, PhD, author of *The How of Happiness: A Scientific Approach to Getting the Life You Want.*

But don't overdo it. Women who kept a gratitude journal only once a week got a bigger boost in happiness than those asked to record their good fortune three times a week. Find the frequency that works for you; giving thanks shouldn't feel like a chore.

THEY'RE RANDOMLY KIND

Do you perform five acts of kindness in any given day? That's the number of good deeds that boosts your sense of well-being and happiness, according to research by Lyubomirsky. Your karmic acts can be minor and unplanned—giving up your seat on the bus or buying an extra latte to give to a coworker. You'll find that the payback greatly exceeds the effort. "You see how much you're appreciated and liked by others," she says.

Be sure to keep up the good work: When Lyubomirsky asked her study subjects to space their five good deeds over the course of a week, the actions started to seem routine and lost some of their therapeutic effects. But don't fret if you can't make the quota daily. "Being spontaneously kind also delivers rewards," she says.

THEY REAPPRAISE THEIR LIVES

Yes, you can rewrite history—and feel better about yourself in the bargain. Set aside a little time each week to write about or record—or even just mentally revisit—an important event in your past. Reflecting on the experience can reshape your perception of it, as well as your expectations for the future, says Robert N. Butler, MD, president of the International Longevity Center-USA in New York City. When creating this "life review," you get to list all your accomplishments, which is an instant self-esteem booster.

Organize your historical review by epochs: your postcollege years, early marriage, career, parenthood. Subdivide each section into triumphs, missteps, and lessons for the future. It's helpful to look at the bad times as well as the good. Perhaps now that a few years have passed, you'll be able to see how that breakup or failed job opportunity opened other doors and finally forgive yourself—and your ex-boyfriend or would-be boss. "Even if a memory is painful, it's good to work through it," says Dr. Butler. "If you can come to terms with past events, you'll be better able to handle tough times down the road."

So be honest, but also go easy on yourself. You are the star of the show.

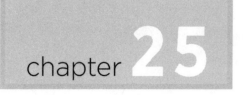

chapter 25

THE STATUS QUOTIENT

Prevent a host of stress-related diseases
with a little social climbing

Picture a ladder with 10 rungs, each representing a higher level of social prestige than the one just below it. At the top of the ladder are the leaders in your community—the good neighbors, parent coaches, Girl Scout leaders, and church elders. At the bottom are the residents who you feel have little status. Now, ask yourself which rung you occupy. You see yourself near the top? Congratulations! The reward for your high self-regard is the promise of a long and healthful life.

You've probably heard that people with big bank accounts and prestigious jobs tend to live longer than those below them on the economic totem pole. Well, similar Rockefeller-like health benefits are also available to the rest of us if we simply do things that enhance our status in our own minds—regardless of our net worth.

"People who perceive themselves as high on the social ladder—regardless of their actual educational degree or size of their paycheck—are less likely to suffer from a range of health problems, including depression, insomnia, and certain risk factors for heart disease," says Nancy Adler, PhD, director of the MacArthur Foundation Research Network on Socio-economic Status and Health. Researchers believe that these people feel more in control of their lives and are better able to cope with stress—and that keeps them healthier.

That's great news, because although you can't exactly ask your boss for a raise on the grounds that it will help you avoid heart disease, you can do some simple things—donate regularly to good causes, be a good role model for your kids—to enhance your sense of self-worth. Make these efforts, and you'll find they add up to a lot more than money in the bank.

"MY COLLEAGUES ARE DOING BETTER THAN I AM"

Move up a rung: Put stock in your reputation.

When you chose your rung on that imaginary ladder, the first thing you did was compare yourself with others. "It's not unusual for us to look around and see how we stack up in a variety of realms—socially, financially, physically, morally," says Joan Ostrove, PhD, an associate professor of psychology at Macalester College. But the individuals you compare yourself with, and what factors you allow into the equation, affect your self-image.

Consider your feelings about your salary. "Part of your satisfaction with your income is based on the reputation you have among people in your field," says Ed Diener, PhD, a psychologist who studies subjective well-being at the University of Illinois. That means you should measure yourself not just by your paycheck but also by your experience and reliability, which make you the go-to person to head up big projects.

Comparing yourself with someone who makes more money can actually boost your self-image—and your productivity—say researchers at Stanford University. The key: placing more emphasis on the ways you're alike than on the ways she outshines you. "If you see that both you and your boss are outgoing and open-minded, for instance, you may feel a sense of kinship, even though there's an income disparity," says Camille Johnson, PhD, lead author of the study and now an assistant professor of management and organizations at San Jose State University.

"I SHOULD BE A BETTER PERSON"

Move up a rung: Be more generous with others.

Our self-image often reflects deeply held principles and standards—and whether we feel we are upholding them. If you're meeting your own ethical goals—you do regular volunteer work, give to worthy causes, and are a responsible parent and thoughtful neighbor—you will likely place yourself high on the community ladder.

In other words, becoming a legend in your own mind may be as simple as offering to help out at the library or heading up a youth outreach group at church. The payoff is substantial: People older than age 55 who volunteer for two or more organizations have half the chance of dying in the next 5 years as those who volunteer with just one group, and they are 63 percent less likely to die in that time than nonvolunteers, according to the Buck Center for Research in Aging in Novato, California.

"Volunteering has as strong an effect on mortality as exercising four times a week," says Stephen Post, PhD, a professor of bioethics at Case Western Reserve University's School of Medicine and coauthor of *Why Good Things Happen to Good People*. "Helping and giving to others increases your self-esteem and gives you a sense of dignity and purpose that enhances your sense of your own status—and, thus, your well-being."

"I'M TOO STRESSED TO CHANGE MY LIFE"

Move up a rung: Seize what control you can.

People who stand lower on the social ladder tend to be under greater stress, researchers have learned. In one study of premenopausal women, Adler found that those who ranked themselves lowest had the highest output of cortisol, a harmful stress hormone, during a 3-day lab experiment in which participants did mental math and other anxiety-provoking activities.

"The women who thought highly of themselves were able to get used to the stress. They released a lot of cortisol the first day, but their levels decreased over the next 2 days," she says. "That didn't happen with the women who said they had low status. They pumped out cortisol throughout the entire experiment."

What's Your Health Status?

People who rank themselves higher on the social ladder have:

A lower resting heart rate

Less abdominal fat

Less frequent insomnia

People who feel they are lower on the social ladder have:

More colds

A shorter life span

A higher prevalence of angina, diabetes, and depression

The bottom line: Minimize stress to improve your health—and your status. Here are three ways to get started:

Keep a good news diary. "Every day, write down five positive things that have happened," suggests Carol Ryff, PhD, director of the Institute on Aging at the University of Wisconsin-Madison. "In order to perceive your life as good, you need to focus on the gratifying things in it."

Stay connected with friends. "You're more likely to feel stressed and have higher cortisol levels if you lack social support," says Robert Sapolsky, PhD, a professor of biology and neurology at Stanford University and author of *Why Zebras Don't Get Ulcers*.

Laugh loud and often. "Laughter prompts the body to secrete natural mood-boosting chemicals and decreases levels of cortisol," says Post. "Keep a drawer full of your favorite comics and cartoons and look at them when you're feeling stressed."

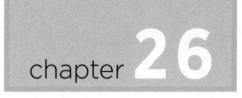

chapter 26

MOOD FOOD

Eat to beat stress: Nine foods that'll keep you jolly

F orget everything you've heard about stress-eating being a bad thing. If you put the right foods in your belly, noshing when your nerves are jangling can actually calm you down. And that's great news, because the last thing you need is more stress, which over time can increase your risk of high blood pressure, heart disease, and obesity—and the odds that you'll go ballistic when a soccer mom driving a land yacht—while talking on the cell phone, gesturing to her kids in the backseat, and sipping on a Starbucks—cuts you off on the highway.

These yummy, easy-to-find foods soothe stress and can counteract the damage that chronic pressure does to your body. Stock up on the lot of them so that when the tension rises—along with the temperature under your collar—you can eat instead of freak.

ALMONDS, PISTACHIOS, AND WALNUTS

When all hell breaks loose, reach for a handful of almonds. They're bursting with vitamin E, which is an antioxidant that bolsters the immune system. Almonds also contain B vitamins, which may help your body hold up during seriously unpleasant events. About a quarter cup every day is all you need. Another easy way to get a fix is to switch from traditional peanut butter to almond butter on high-tension days. (We like All Natural Barney Butter Almond Butter, $7, www.barneybutter.com.)

Sick of almonds? Shell pistachios or crack walnuts. Both will help keep your heart from racing when things heat up. "We experience immediate cardiovascular responses to stress because of the 'fight or flight' response," says Sheila G. West, MD, associate professor of biobehavioral health at Pennsylvania State University. When stress strikes, the hormone adrenaline raises blood pressure to boost energy—so you're prepared to run like hell if you need to. But because we seldom need to fight or flee (dodging road rage–crazed drivers doesn't count), it's better to blunt the strain on your heart. A 2007 Penn State study led by Dr. West found that eating $1\frac{1}{2}$ ounces (about a handful) of pistachios a day lowers blood pressure so your heart doesn't have to work overtime. Walnuts have also been found to lower blood pressure, both at rest and under stress, Dr. West says. Add about an ounce to salads, cereal, or oatmeal.

AVOCADOS

The next time stress has you hankering for a high-fat, creamy treat, skip the ice cream and try some homemade guacamole. The thick, rich texture can satisfy your craving and reduce those frantic feelings. Plus, the green wonder's double whammy of monounsaturated fat and potassium can lower blood pressure.

One of the best ways to reduce high blood pressure, according to the National Heart, Lung, and Blood Institute, is to get enough potassium—and just half an avocado offers 487 milligrams, more than you'll get from a medium-size banana. To whip up your own avocado salad dressing, purée a medium avocado with 2 tablespoons of lemon juice and a dash of cayenne pepper.

FAT-FREE MILK

Science backs up the old warm-milk remedy for insomnia and restlessness. Turns out calcium can reduce muscle spasms and soothe tension, says Mary Dallman, PhD, professor of physiology at the University of California, San Francisco. A glass of moo juice (preferably fat-free or 1 percent) may also reduce stressful symptoms such as mood swings, anxiety, and irritability. According to a 2005 study from the *Archives of Internal Medicine*, women who drank four or more servings of low-fat or fat-free milk per day had a 46 percent lower risk of pre-period misery than women who had no more than one serving per week.

OATMEAL

Carbohydrates make the brain produce more serotonin, the same relaxing brain chemical released when you eat dark chocolate. The more slowly your body absorbs carbs, the more steadily serotonin flows, according to Judith Wurtman, PhD, a former MIT research scientist and coauthor of *The Serotonin Power Diet*. The result: a less-likely-to-snap you. Because thick, hearty oatmeal is high in fiber, few things take longer for your stomach to digest, says Elizabeth Somer, RD, author of *Food & Mood*.

Wurtman also recommends topping it with a swirl of jam for a quicker release of serotonin. When you know it's going to be a doozy of a day, avoid heavily processed varieties (e.g., the sugary kind that comes in packets meant for the microwave), which are digested more quickly, and take the time to make thick-cut old-fashioned oats, such as McCann's Original Steel-Cut Irish Oatmeal ($6 for 28 ounces, www.amazon.com). But if 2 minutes for breakfast is all you have, you can still do your mood a favor by opting for instant oatmeal over Cocoa Puffs.

ORANGES

Fretting over a job interview or presentation at work? Pour yourself a glass of Florida's famous juice or peel yourself an orange. The magic nutrient here is vitamin C. In a study in *Psychopharmacology*, German researchers subjected 120 people to a public-speaking task plus a series of math problems. Those who took 3,000 milligrams of vitamin C reported that they felt less stressed, and their blood pressure and levels of cortisol (a stress hormone) returned to normal faster.

Mellow Menu

Here's a day's worth of stress-busting meals.

Breakfast: Top plain oatmeal with slivered almonds (a golf ball-size serving), dried cranberries (dried fruit offers all the health benefits of regular fruit), and a splash of DHA-fortified low-fat milk. Wash it down with an 8-ounce glass of Tropicana Healthy Heart with Omega-3 orange juice.

Snack: Munch on pistachio popcorn to satisfy sweet, salty, and nutty cravings: Top a Pop Secret 100 Calorie Pop pack with 2 tablespoons of shelled pistachios and a sprinkling of vanilla extract.

Lunch: Build your own stress-battling BLT—toast whole wheat bread and stack on about a cup of spinach, a strip or two of crispy turkey bacon, and tomato slices. To drink, have an iced OJ spritzer (half orange juice, half sparkling mineral water).

Snack: Toast a Kellogg's Eggo Nutri-Grain Low Fat Whole Wheat waffle and top it with a tablespoon of almond butter.

Dinner: Have grilled salmon topped with avocado tomato salsa (add a quarter of an avocado, cubed, to your favorite salsa) on a bed of fresh spinach.

Snack: Indulge in three squares of an Endangered Species Chocolate Dark Chocolate with Blueberries bar and a glass of low-fat milk ($3.15, www.chocolatebar.com).

"Vitamin C is also a well-known immune system booster," says Amy Jamieson-Petonic, RD, a spokesperson for the American Dietetic Association.

SALMON

Stress hormones have an archenemy: omega-3 fatty acids. A 2003 study from *Diabetes & Metabolism* found that a diet rich in omega-3 fatty acids kept cortisol and adrenaline from geysering. Omega-3 fatty acids also protect against heart disease, according to a 2002 study in the *Journal of the American Medical Association*.

"Eat a 3-ounce serving of fish, especially fatty fish like salmon, mackerel, herring, and light tuna, at least twice a week," Jamieson-Petonic says. Not a fish eater? For another omega-3 punch, buy foods fortified with DHA. (You'll find this particular fatty acid in eggs, yogurt, milk, and soy products.) But don't go out of your way for products that boast booming levels of ALA, another fatty acid, which may not work as well.

SPINACH

Magnesium was made to calm insanity. First, the mineral can help lower your stress levels, keeping your body in a state of relative ease as you kick off yet another round of small talk at the company party. Not getting enough magnesium may trigger migraine headaches and make you feel fatigued. (And almost 7 out of 10 of us don't get enough of the stuff. No wonder we're cranky.) Just 1 cup of spinach provides 40 percent of your daily value. Try subbing it for lettuce on sandwiches and salads. (And now you have an excuse to indulge in the spinach dip at said party!)

part
6

AVOID COMPLICATIONS

medical
BREAKTHROUGHS

Diabetes brings along with it many unwanted complications, such as dental problems, heart issues, and cancer. Here's the latest research on some of these unwelcome tag-a-longs.

SAVE YOUR LIFE WITH DENTAL FLOSS

People with diabetes need to pay close attention to their mouths. Spanish researchers studied 20 people with gum disease, characterized by puffy red gums. Half of them had diabetes. All the volunteers underwent scaling and root planing—the standard dental treatment. Afterward, the blood sugar levels of the people with diabetes dropped by as much as 20 percent and remained down for at least 3 months, significantly reducing their risk of complications such as heart disease, stroke, and kidney failure.

Researchers say that for people with diabetes, it's especially critical to brush after every meal, floss at least once a day—preferably at night—and see a dentist regularly.

WATCH YOUR CARBS

People with diabetes know that eating too many "bad carbs" is bad for blood sugar. They may be surprised to learn, however, that it can have disastrous consequences for your vision as well. Scientists at Tufts University studied 3,400 people and found that those who ate the most candy, crackers, and other troublesome carbs were 29 percent more likely to have the most common type of lens-clouding cataracts than those who ate the fewest. And in a study of 526 people, the scientists found that eating lots of refined carbs raised by 170 percent the risk of age-related macular degeneration (AMD), which is a leading cause of blindness in the United States.

Here's why. Experts say that bad carbs cause blood sugar spikes, which trigger a damaging process in the eye called sugar oxidation. This is even more reason why people with diabetes should limit their intake of refined carbs and switch to healthier carbs such as whole-grain bread and cereals.

B CAREFUL

People with diabetes could have a dangerous vitamin deficiency. When British researchers analyzed blood plasma from people with type 1 or type 2 diabetes, they discovered that levels of the B vitamin thiamine were 75 percent lower than normal. Thiamine may help protect blood vessels from the damaging effects of high glucose levels, so the deficiency may be partly responsible for the spikes in heart attack and stroke risk associated with diabetes, says JoAnn Manson, MD, a Harvard endocrinologist. One caution: Doctors usually use red blood cells to measure thiamine, but recent research shows that this method may be unreliable. Make sure your doctor checks your thiamine level by using your plasma instead.

RAISE A GLASS

Think diabetes is muddying your thinking? It's not your imagination. Particularly in older adults, diabetes causes memory problems and difficulty understanding things.

One thing you might not expect would *help* this problem is a little alcohol. But it turns out it just might. Researchers at Massachusetts General Hospital and Harvard Medical School, both in Boston, compared people with diabetes who drank up to two drinks a day with people who didn't drink alcohol at all. The researchers discovered that the drinker group performed better on three of five cognitive tests than the abstainer group did.

BREATHE UNEASY

Even lung function may be impaired when you have diabetes. Researchers at the Johns Hopkins University in Maryland sought to test the theory that diabetes is associated with changes in lung function. They studied 1,100 people with diabetes and 10,162 people without diabetes, checking their diabetes status and forced vital capacity (FVC), which is a measure of lung function, at the beginning of the study and 3 years later.

The researchers discovered that at the beginning of the study, the people with diabetes had significantly lower FVC than the people without diabetes. As the study progressed, the people with diabetes experienced a faster decline in FVC than the people without diabetes.

The researchers concluded that the lung is a target organ for diabetic injury.

DODGE ALZHEIMER'S DISEASE

As we mentioned earlier, people with diabetes have an increased risk of problems with cognitive thinking. But no one knows why. In an attempt to puzzle it out, researchers in Sweden reviewed data from a study called the Uppsala Longitudinal Study of Adult Men, which began in 1970 when the 2,322 volunteers were 50 years old. At that time, researchers checked the volunteer's insulin response and glucose tolerance, which are two measures of blood sugar control. After 32 years had passed, 102 of the men had been diagnosed with Alzheimer's disease.

The researchers discovered that a low response to insulin at the beginning of the study was associated with a higher risk of Alzheimer's disease at the end of the study, which suggests a causal link between insulin metabolism and Alzheimer's disease.

People with diabetes might consider following suggestions from the Alzheimer's Association to prevent the disease, such as staying mentally, physically, and socially active and eating a brain-healthy diet that includes plenty of antioxidant-rich fruits and vegetables, omega-3 fatty-acid–rich fish, and vitamin E-rich nuts.

FIGHT PSORIASIS

Dastardly diabetes can even wreak havoc with your skin. Studies in the past have shown a relationship between metabolic syndrome and psoriasis, but there have been only a few studies on the link between diabetes and psoriasis. So researchers in Israel sought to study the relationship between them.

The scientists studied 16,851 people with psoriasis and 74,987 people without psoriasis. They found that the people with psoriasis were more likely to have diabetes than the people without psoriasis, no matter what their age or gender was.

The researchers suggested that people with psoriasis take care to reduce risk factors, such as reducing blood pressure and not smoking.

KICK BUTT

Smoking is no good for anyone, and certainly not anyone with diabetes. Here's one more reason why: The deadly sticks exacerbate nephropathy, a type of kidney disease. And quitting smoking eases it.

Researchers at Texas Tech University Health Sciences Center, Scott and White Memorial Hospital, and the Texas A&M Health Sciences Center College of Medicine studied 91 people with diabetes—39 who smoked and 52 who didn't. The smokers received help to try to quit, and 11 of them were successful. The researchers discovered that smoking exacerbated the progression of early kidney disease to advanced, but quitting smoking protected the kidneys when kidney disease was still in an early stage.

BE HEART SMART

Diabetes can be a real heart breaker. Even though the past 50 years has seen a marked drop in the number of people affected by heart disease, the same can't be said for people with diabetes. Researchers of the National Heart, Lung, and Blood Institute's Framington Heart Study compared people who were studied during the "early" years of the Framington Heart Study (1952 to 1974) with people who were studied during the "late" years of the study (1975 to 1998).

The researchers discovered that, unlike in the rest of the population, the proportion of cardiovascular disease attributable to diabetes has increased over the past half century. The researchers concluded that people with diabetes need to be especially vigilant in controlling their risk factors for heart disease.

Here are five simple ways to keep your heart healthy, from the Mayo Clinic:

- If you smoke, quit
- Get 30 to 60 minutes of exercise most days of the week
- Eat a heart-healthy diet rich in fruits, vegetables, whole grains, and low-fat dairy
- Maintain a healthy weight
- Get regular health screenings, such as blood pressure and cholesterol checks

LOVE YOUR DOVE

Regularly eating a small amount of dark chocolate lowers blood pressure, reports the *Journal of the American Medical Association*. Forty-four people with slightly elevated blood pressure ate a daily dose of 30 calories of dark or white chocolate. After 18 weeks, the dark-chocolate eaters' blood pressure had dropped an average of 3 points; white-chocolate eaters experienced no change. Chemicals called polyphenols in cocoa may widen blood vessels, decreasing blood pressure, says researcher Dirk Taubert, MD, PhD. Look for bars with a cocoa content of at least 40 to 50 percent.

Another study, this one conducted by researchers in Turkey, found that a higher intake of black tea, fruits, and vegetables protected people with diabetes from developing high blood pressure.

SAY SOY LONG HIGH BLOOD PRESSURE

A snack that could slash blood pressure: soy nuts. Postmenopausal women who replaced half of their daily protein intake with ½ cup of soy nuts cut their systolic blood pressure by as much as 5.2 percent over 8 weeks. Those with hypertension saw even bigger benefits. Their blood pressure decreased up to twice as much, and their low-density lipoprotein (LDL) cholesterol (the "bad" cholesterol) level dropped by 11 percent.

To liven up the taste without adding many calories (½ cup of plain soy nuts has 240), toss nuts in a zipper-lock bag, lightly spritz with cooking spray, and sprinkle with salt-free Cajun seasoning or apple pie spice. Shake and eat!

STRETCH YOUR HEART HEALTHY

Here's a good reason to loosen up daily: The more easily you can touch your toes, the lower your blood pressure and heart disease risk are likely to be, reveals a Japanese study. The most limber over-40 women had about 7 percent less arterial stiffness (a marker of heart disease) then their less-flexible peers. Increased bloodflow from stretching may expand arteries, keeping them pliable. For your healthiest heart, continue doing cardio, but stretch for 5 to 10 minutes afterward when muscles are warm.

chapter 27

THE HEART ATTACK PREVENTION PLAN

Focus on your cardiovascular system
to keep the beat going on

Father Time is a sneaky little guy. As we age, camouflaging it every step of the way with moisturizers, hair dye, and other lotions and potions, he's wreaking unseen havoc deep inside of us. Here are a few of his hasty tricks.

Cholesterol levels shift. High-density lipoprotein (HDL) cholesterol (the "good" cholesterol) sweeps up low-density lipoprotein (LDL) cholesterol (the "bad" cholesterol) and shunts it to the liver for removal. Without enough HDL, the bad stuff builds up, causing plaque.

Plaque causes clots. Plaque is a mix of fatty substances, including LDL cholesterol, which burrows into and inflames artery walls. When a plaque deposit bursts, the body's healing mechanism produces a clot. This can obstruct the artery and cause a heart attack.

Arteries become weak and stiff. High blood pressure hardens flexible arteries, which strains the heart, rips open plaque deposits, and promotes blood vessel leaks that can

Protect Your Heart Like the Mediterraneans ─────

Olive oil, leafy greens, whole grains, nuts, fruit, fish, red wine, tomatoes—their rich blend of antioxidants, phytochemicals, vitamins, and healthy fats cuts cardiovascular risks. Just 3 months of Mediterranean-style eating in one recent study improved blood sugar, blood pressure, and cholesterol in people at high risk of heart disease.

The Mediterranean diet offers good sources of chromium, which may lower bad and raise good cholesterol as well as prevent insulin resistance (the hallmark of diabetes), but it's hard to get enough of the mineral from food. Best bet: Take a daily multivitamin with chromium.

---

cause an aneurysm or stroke. Blood vessels are lined with the same kind of tissue as your skin. "It's just as important to keep your inner skin as beautiful as the visible skin," says Lori Mosca, MD, PhD, an associate professor of medicine at Columbia University in New York City. "Instead of protecting it from the sun, you need to prevent damage from a poor diet or lack of exercise."

Blood can become "sticky." High blood sugar is like a soda spill on a counter-top—it permits plaque-forming material to fasten more easily to artery walls. It's also a symptom of diabetes, which doubles your risk of heart disease or stroke.

Waist size expands. Slowing metabolism leads to weight gain, which contributes to diabetes, high blood pressure, and high cholesterol. "Large waist size is the most important risk factor. It compounds all the others," says Annabelle Volgman, MD, medical director of the Heart Center for Women at Rush University Medical Center in Chicago.

YOUR STAY-YOUNG PLAN

Fortunately, there are things you can do to outwit Father Time, or at least slow him down.

Keep moving. "Physical activity reduces every controllable risk factor," says Dr. Volg-man. Just 10 minutes of cardiovascular exercise on most days can cut a sedentary person's heart attack risk in half.

Do intervals. By boosting aerobic fitness and metabolism, twice-a-week interval training (short bursts of high-intensity exercise) for just 2 weeks can reduce heart disease risks by 20 percent, according to studies. Get started: Simply vary the pace of your daily walk for 2 minutes every 10.

Number of heartbeats in the average lifetime: 2.5 billion

Monitor your markers. Keep a copy of the blood work you have done during your annual physical and track changes over time. Make sure your numbers are always within these ranges:

Cholesterol: LDL under 100 milligrams per deciliter (mg/dL); HDL above 45 (men) and 55 (women)

Blood pressure: Below 130/80 millimeters of mercury (mm Hg)

Fasting blood sugar: Less than 100 mg/dL

Triglycerides: Less than 150 mg/dL

Get "subclass" cholesterol tests. If you have heart disease or are at risk, ask for a test called lipoprotein subfraction, which measures the size of your cholesterol particles. If your LDL particles are very small, they are better able to burrow into artery walls; despite normal or low cholesterol readings, you may need more-aggressive monitoring and treatment.

Test for inflammation. Doctors now know that when LDL cholesterol damages the arterial wall, the artery becomes chronically inflamed, starting a cascade of events that may culminate in a heart attack. As part of this inflammatory response, your body produces a substance called C-reactive protein (CRP), which can be measured in a blood test. If you have normal cholesterol but a high level of CRP, you may need a more aggressive preventive plan (more-intense monitoring of lipids).

(continued on page 226)

Quick Tip

Have a truffle for dessert. Eating a 30-calorie dark chocolate daily for 2 weeks will lower systolic blood pressure by 3 points and diastolic pressure by 2.

Nature's Heart Healers

Make room in your pantry for a new batch of disease-fighting products: foods fortified with sterols and stanols, plant compounds proven to protect your heart. Sterols and stanols are found naturally in fruits, vegetables, nuts, and oils. Adding 2 grams of either to your daily diet can help lower your total cholesterol by about 10 percent—often within 2 weeks, according to numerous studies published in both American and European medical journals. That may not sound like a substantial reduction, but it could translate to a 20 percent lower risk of heart disease, which is the number one killer in the United States, says Joseph Keenan, MD, a professor of family medicine and a joint professor of food science and nutrition at the University of Minnesota.

Our primer will help you better understand how these unique compounds work, how they can protect your health, and the easiest way to incorporate them into your diet.

For more than 5 decades, scientists have known about the health benefits of these compounds, but natural foods don't provide a high enough concentration to budge your cholesterol. (A tablespoon of corn oil, the best natural source, has only 0.13 gram of sterols; that's a long way to go to reach the recommended 2 grams a day.) But in the 1980s, Finnish chemists found a way to extract the sterols and stanols from plants and add them to the fat in foods. These new compounds, called sterol and stanol esters, first cropped up in margarine-type spreads in 2000. Today, new technology allows researchers to extract them from different plants and fortify more foods—such as cheese, orange juice, breads, and milk. Popular sterol brands you'll find in foods include Cardio-Aid (made by food manufacturer Archer Daniels Midland) and Coro-Wise (made by Cargill). In 2008, global market researchers predict sterol-fortified products will be a $250 million industry, nearly three times what it was when such products first hit supermarket shelves.

How do they work? Plant sterols and stanols act much like cholesterol itself: Soft and waxy, they serve as building blocks for hormones, vitamins, and cell walls. These structural similarities give them their cholesterol-lowering capabilities. As sterols travel through the digestive tract, they compete with cholesterol, so some of the sterols are absorbed into the bloodstream instead of artery-clogging cholesterol. The bonus: Studies show that sterols and stanols don't affect artery-protecting HDL cholesterol.

Who needs them? Sterols are most helpful when your cholesterol levels are slightly high (200 to 239 total cholesterol, 130 to 159 LDL). If your levels are substantially elevated

(240 or higher total, 160 or higher LDL), your doctor will help determine if sterols, cholesterol-lowering medication (statins), or a combination of the two is best. Studies have shown that together, sterols and statins are more effective than taking a double dose of cholesterol-lowering medications. They're an especially good choice for avoiding drug side effects. "If one of my patients has a high LDL level but doesn't tolerate statin drugs well, I recommend plant sterols and plenty of fiber," says Arthur Agatston, MD, a preventive cardiologist and an assistant professor of medicine at the University of Miami Miller School of Medicine.

If your cholesterol is healthy (less than 200 total, less than 100 LDL), adding sterols to your diet won't hurt, but the cholesterol reductions will not be as great, says Cyril Kendall, PhD, a research scientist at the University of Toronto who has studied plant sterols for the past 7 years.

Who should avoid them? Scientists don't know if sterol- and stanol-fortified foods are safe for pregnant women and children, so it's best if these groups skip them altogether. Also important to note: Initial research indicates that sterols can interfere with the absorption of some carotenoids, such as beta-carotene, which your body uses to make vitamin A. If you eat sterols, include a few servings of vegetables rich in beta-carotene—such as carrots, squash, sweet potatoes, and dark leafy greens—to your diet once or twice a week to compensate, suggests Dr. Keenan.

How do you eat them? Stick to 2 grams a day; getting more may actually reduce the positive effects, says Dr. Kendall. And once you start eating sterol-fortified foods, don't stop—otherwise your LDL levels will head back up. Follow the following guidelines.

Split up your 2-grams-daily goal. "Have about 1 gram at breakfast and then another at either lunch or dinner," says Dr. Keenan. This helps prevent absorption of the cholesterol in your meal and also blocks the cholesterol your body manufactures during digestion—which amounts to about 80 percent of your total count.

Use them as substitutes. If a food you already eat comes in a sterol-fortified version, use that product instead. Otherwise, try to cut an equivalent number of calories elsewhere in your diet. Because sterol-fortified foods aren't necessarily low cal, they may cause harmful weight gain if you aren't mindful of how much you're eating.

(*continued*)

Nature's Heart Healers (*cont.*)

Include them as part of a low-fat, low-cholesterol, high-fiber diet. That will reduce your risk of heart disease even more. Although sterols and stanols do give your heart a boost, they aren't your only route to good health. (See "Moves to Cut LDL 30 Percent" below for ideal eating rules for your heart.)

For an extended list of sterol-fortified foods and a sample cholesterol-cutting menu and to create and print a customized grocery list, visit www.prevention.com/heartsmartfoods.

Moves to Cut LDL 30 Percent

According to the National Institutes of Health's Cholesterol Education Program, try the following tips to reduce your LDL.

Reduce saturated fat to less than 7 percent of calories. (For a 2,000-calorie diet, that's less than 15.5 grams.)

Control calories to help maintain a healthy weight.

Decrease dietary cholesterol to less than 200 milligrams per day.

Have 20 to 30 grams of fiber per day (10 to 25 grams should be soluble fiber).

Add 2 grams of sterols/stanols per day.

Nature's Top 10

Fortified products may offer a heftier dose, but the following natural foods have some sterols, plus other benefits.

Corn oil: It's a good source of healthy polyunsaturated fat, which helps cut cholesterol. 0.13 gram* per 1 tablespoon

Sunflower oil: High in monounsaturated fat, it lowers the risk of heart disease and provides nutrients to keep cells healthy. 0.1 gram per 1 tablespoon

Beans: They're full of fiber; studies show that fiber-rich foods help lower your heart attack risk. 0.07 gram per ½ cup

Corn: It contains folate, a B vitamin that reduces damage to blood vessels. 0.06 gram per ½ cup

Peanut butter: The protein keeps you feeling full, which helps keep weight in check. 0.05 gram per 2 tablespoons

---

*Amount of natural sterols present

Olive oil: An excellent source of good monounsaturated fats, which help lower bad LDL cholesterol and raise good HDL cholesterol. 0.03 gram per 1 tablespoon

Almonds: The monounsaturated fats and vitamin E work together to cut cholesterol. 0.02 gram per 1 ounce

Oranges: This fruit is an excellent source of immune-boosting vitamin C. 0.02 gram per 1 small

Apples: They provide filling, waist-friendly fiber. 0.01 gram per 1 small

Avocados: Known for their monounsaturated fat, they also contain potassium to help regulate blood pressure. 0.008 gram per 1 ounce

Sterols at the Supermarket

The National Institutes of Health advises getting 2 grams daily of plant sterols and stanols from fortified foods such as the following to lower your cholesterol.

Dairy Aisle

Promise Activ Super Shots (serving size: 3 ounces)

    Sterol: 2 grams

    Calories: 70

    Fat: 3.5 grams (0 grams sat fat)

    Fiber: Less than 1 gram

Lifetime Low Fat Block Cheddar (serving size: 1 ounce)

    Sterol: 0.65 gram

    Calories: 55

    Fat: 2.5 grams (1 gram sat fat)

    Fiber: 1 gram

Lifetime Low Fat Cheese Singles (serving size: 1 slice)

    Sterol: 0.65 gram

    Calories: 30

    Fat: 1 gram (0.5 gram sat fat)

    Fiber: 0 grams

(*continued*)

Nature's Heart Healers (*cont.*) ———————

Kroger Active Lifestyle Fat Free Milk (serving size: 8 ounces)

Sterol: 0.4 gram

Calories: 90

Fat: 0 grams

Fiber: 0 grams

Juices and drinks

CocoaVia Rich Chocolate Indulgence Beverage (serving size: 5.65 ounces)

Sterol: 1.1 grams

Calories: 150

Fat: 3 grams (1 gram sat fat)

Fiber: 3 grams

Minute Maid Premium Heart Wise Orange Juice (serving size: 8 ounces)

Sterol: 1 gram

Calories: 110

Fat: 0 grams

Fiber: Less than 1 gram

Rice Dream Heartwise Vanilla Rice Milk (serving size: 8 ounces)

Sterol: 0.65 gram

Calories: 140

Fat: 2 grams

Fiber: 3 grams

Bread

Thomas' Hearty Grains Oatmeal and Honey English Muffins (serving size: 1 muffin)

Sterol: 0.4 gram

Calories: Up to 290

Fat: Up to 2 grams (up to 0.5 gram sat fat)

Fiber: Up to 3 grams

Vitamuffin Dark Chocolate Pomegranate Vita Top (serving size: 1 muffin top)

Sterol: 0.4 gram

Calories: 100

Fat: 1.5 grams (0.5 gram sat fat)

Fiber: 6 grams

Snacks

Right Direction Cookies (serving size: 1 cookie)

Sterol: 1.3 grams

Calories: Up to 150

Fat: Up to 6 grams (up to 2 grams sat fat)

Fiber: Up to 6 grams

CocoaVia Chocolate Covered Almonds (serving size: 1 ounce)

Sterol: 1.1 grams

Calories: 140

Fat: 11 grams (3.5 grams sat fat)

Fiber: 3 grams

Nature Valley Healthy Heart Chewy Honey-Nut Granola Bar (serving size: 1 bar)

Sterol: 0.4 gram

Calories: 160

Fat: 4 grams (0.5 gram sat fat)

Fiber: 3 grams

Corazonas Tortilla Chips (serving size: 1 ounce)

Sterol: 0.4 gram

Calories: 140

Fat: 7 grams (0.5 gram sat fat)

Fiber: 3 grams

Screen out false positives. Make sure to ask for the high-sensitivity test, which rules out other causes of inflammation, such as infection, injury, and arthritis.

Brush your teeth, clean your arteries. Cutting your risk of heart disease may be as easy as regularly flossing and brushing. Columbia University doctors have found that people whose mouths contain a high number of the bacteria that cause gum disease are more likely to have plaque-clogged arteries.

Save every tooth. Keep an eye out for gum recession. A recent study found that men ages 40 to 75 who had lost eight or more teeth because of gum disease had a 57 percent higher risk of stroke than those who had lost less than eight.

Get a baseline heart scan. Prominent cardiologists recommend that women older than age 50 who are postmenopausal and have any risk factors for coronary disease get a heart scan—several different technologies are available—to measure coronary artery calcium, which directly correlates to the total amount of plaque in your arteries. An early baseline enables your doctor to monitor signs of heart disease.

Get a highly detailed picture. Opt for the brand-new 64-slice computed tomography (CT) scanner, which measures calcium and the amount of dangerous soft plaque in the arteries. Filled primarily with cholesterol, soft plaque is prone to rupture, resulting in a blood clot that can cause a heart attack.

ON THE CUTTING EDGE

Here are the five newest heart attack fighters, according to the American Heart Association's new prevention guidelines for women.

Eat more omega-3 fatty acids. They curb inflammation, lower blood pressure, and slow plaque growth. To get more, eat oily fish such as salmon at least twice a week and consider taking Eicosapentaenoic acid (EPA) and docosahexaenoic (DHA) supplements of 850 to 1,000 mg a day if you have heart disease.

Take aspirin with a doctor's okay. Low doses prevent clots that cause heart attacks, but regular use can cause stomach bleeding and increased stroke risk. "Whether you should take it depends on your age and family history," says Dr. Mosca.

Avoid antioxidant supplements. Recent research suggests that high doses of beta-carotene, vitamin A, and vitamin E may increase the risk of premature death, and too much vitamin C may boost the risk of dying for women over age 50 with diabetes.

Cut saturated fat even further. Artery-damaging fat should account for less than 10 percent of daily calories. Ideally, you should keep it below 7 percent. Be vigilant about reading food labels to avoid eating partially hydrogenated (trans) fats.

Trim 200 calories a day after menopause. After 50, your metabolism slows about 5 percent a decade, so your body burns less energy even if you're moderately active.

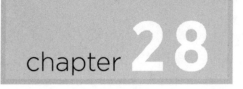

chapter **28**

HIGH BLOOD
PRESSURE HELP

20 ways to soothe your raging veins

f you were an airline pilot, chances are you wouldn't feel safe flying with the plane's gauges pegged in the red zone. Oh, you could taxi down the runway, take off, and probably remain airborne for a spell. You might even stay up long enough to enjoy an in-flight meal. But the expectation of eventually seeing smoke billowing from the engines, or hearing shards of metal snap off, would fill you with dread.

Strange, then, that most people don't sweat it when their body's most important gauge—blood pressure—rises into the red zone and stays there. "High blood pressure gives you a twofold to fourfold increase in your risk of stroke or heart attack," says Prediman K. Shah, MD, director of cardiology at Cedars-Sinai Medical Center in Los Angeles. "And only about one-third of individuals with high blood pressure have it under some sort of control."

The problem is, most of us mistake the early stages of hypertension for completely normal blood pressure. In the past few years, 120/80 millimeters of mercury (mm Hg) went

Off-the-Cuff Advice

An inaccurate blood pressure reading can cause more trouble than no reading at all—and everything from your shirtsleeve to your last meal and how you sit can skew the score. Follow these tips for a true measure.

Shed your outer layers. Nurses and doctors don't always ask you to take off your shirt before measuring your blood pressure, but wearing a sweatshirt or bulky sweater could lead to an artificially raised reading. Thick sleeves boosted systolic pressure measurements by as much as 22 mm Hg in people with high blood pressure in a Tel Aviv University study. Dress shirts and thin sweaters are fine; a study in the journal *Blood Pressure* revealed that measurements taken over bare skin were the same as those taken through sleeves less than 2 mm thick.

Elevate your arm to heart level. The blood pressure guidelines set forth by the National Heart, Lung, and Blood Institute are based on measurements taken from people holding their arms at heart level. Most doctors and nurses slap the cuff on your arm when it's resting on a desk or chair, which can raise both diastolic and systolic pressure by 6 to 9 points, according to a study by Dutch researchers.

Sit for 16. In a study published in the *American Journal of Hypertension*, researchers discovered that patients who sat for 16 minutes before having their blood pressure checked received more-accurate readings than those who sat for less time. When you stand or move around, your blood vessels constrict, and the longer you sit, the more time they have to return to normal size, lowering blood pressure.

Hit the bathroom. Holding back your bladder can artificially raise your blood pressure reading by making your nervous system think you're stressed.

Avoid finger cuffs. All our experts panned finger cuffs. "The closer to your trunk, the more accurate monitors become," says John Elefteriades, MD, chief of cardiothoracic surgery at Yale. Finger cuffs are also susceptible to shifts in body temperature and finger position.

from being classified as healthy to being "prehypertensive" by the National Heart, Lung, and Blood Institute. The target numbers are now 119/79 mm Hg or lower. For people with diabetes, it's usually 130/80 mm Hg. To hit that target, and avoid a crash landing, let the steam out of the following "pressure cookers" one at a time.

EXCESS BAGGAGE AROUND YOUR GUT

Your heart and the 60,000 miles of veins, arteries, and capillaries in your body have enough work to do when you're lean. Don't make matters worse by adding a beer belly, which requires more blood supply, putting additional strain on the heart and raising overall blood pressure.

"It's infrequent that people are rail thin yet have high blood pressure," says Eric Topol, MD, chief academic officer of Scripps Health. "By bringing your weight into line with what it should be, you can produce a 10- to 29-point drop in blood pressure," says John Elefteriades, MD, chief of cardiothoracic surgery at Yale. For people with borderline high blood pressure, that alone is enough of a drop to eliminate the need for pharmaceutical intervention, he says.

Do this: Eat meat. In a recent Australian study, people with high blood pressure who replaced 8 percent of their daily calories from bread, cereal, potatoes, or pasta with lean red meat experienced a 4-point drop in their systolic blood pressure in just 8 weeks. Arginine, an amino acid in red meat, may help dilate blood vessels, lowering blood pressure. Plus, limiting starches lowers blood sugar and makes your body more efficient at burning fat.

Not that: Eat a low-fat diet. Removing fat from your diet could actually work against your goal, because healthy fats are key to lowering blood pressure. For example, a study in the *Journal of Medicinal Food* found that people who replaced their regular cooking oil with sesame oil for 45 days experienced decreases in their blood pressure and blood sugar. Sesame oil contains polyunsaturated fatty acids and a compound called sesamin, which stops your liver from making cholesterol. Look in the ingredient list on your salad dressing bottle for sesame oil. We like Annie's Naturals Organic Asian Sesame Dressing, which also contains heart-healthy garlic.

INACTIVITY

"You can achieve up to a 10-point drop in blood pressure from regular aerobic exercise," says Dr. Elefteriades. A solid workout raises your blood pressure, which gives your body practice in bringing it back down. Well-trained blood vessels expand and contract easily, which helps control blood pressure, even during times of heightened or prolonged stress.

Do this: Simply squeeze a rubber ball. It seems to help—a lot, actually. According to a study in the *European Journal of Applied Physiology*, people performing handgrip exercises for 8 weeks lowered their systolic blood pressure by 15 points and their diastolic pressure by 5. "The blood pressure response to grip training is greater than to aerobic exercise," says lead author Maureen MacDonald, PhD. All it takes is 2 minutes of squeezing, four times a day.

Not that: Train like a hamster running around in a wheel. Overdosing on cardio can limit the benefits your gym session has on your blood vessels, so add resistance training to the mix. Researchers at the University of Michigan found that people who performed three total body weight workouts a week for 2 months lowered their blood pressure readings by an average of 8 points.

THE BOTTLE

This is a case of too much of a good thing. "Once you exceed two alcoholic beverages a day, you begin to incur complications, such as an increased risk of high blood pressure," says Dr. Shah. No one is quite sure why an excessive amount of alcohol, which dilates blood vessels, can sometimes raise blood pressure, but it does. No need for you to become as dry as a Steven Wright punch line, though. In fact, Harvard researchers recently analyzed the drinking habits of 11,000 men with high blood pressure and determined that those who consumed two drinks a day were 30 percent less likely to have a heart attack than those who drank less.

Do this: Make it a Bloody Mary. According to a study in the *American Heart Journal*, the antioxidant lycopene in tomato juice can boost your beverage's blood pressure–lowering power. When participants in the study swallowed tomato juice extract for 8 weeks, they experienced a 10-point drop in their systolic blood pressure and a 4-point fall in their diastolic measure. Add a stalk of celery for extra protection. High in fiber, celery has been used for centuries in Asian medicine to drop blood pressure.

Not that: Drink on an empty stomach. Keep your bar tab in check, and don't drink any alcoholic beverage without eating something along with it. Researchers at the State University of New York at Buffalo found that a man's risk of high blood pressure increases nearly 50 percent if he boozes between meals. Eating while you imbibe may slow you down and help limit the total amount of alcohol you ingest, the researchers say.

SALT

The white stuff causes your body to retain water, which increases blood volume and, consequently, blood pressure. The results are deadly: The more sodium you eat, the shorter your life, according to researchers at the University of Helsinki. They reviewed more than a dozen studies and found that people who reduced their sodium intake by 30 percent lived an average of 7 years longer than those whose sodium intake remained high. (The national average is over 4,000 milligrams a day—1,600 milligrams more than is recommended.)

Do this: Mix up a DIY salt substitute. Australian scientists determined that diluting regular salt with potassium salt and Epsom salt lowers arterial blood pressure by 6 points. Cooking with the concoction reduces overall sodium intake and boosts blood levels of potassium, which is a nutrient that naturally regulates blood pressure. Pour 65 percent table salt, 25 percent Morton Salt Substitute (potassium chloride), and 10 percent Epsom salt into a small bowl, mix well, and funnel into a saltshaker. You won't taste the difference.

Not that: Skip the saltshaker altogether. You need some sodium in your diet to survive. (One recent study revealed that too little of the mineral can actually increase your risk of death by 37 percent.) Instead, focus on eliminating supersources of salt, such as processed foods. One frozen dinner can contain as much as 2,000 milligrams of sodium, a cup of cottage cheese packs 918 milligrams, and a single slice of deli ham packs 240 milligrams.

Partners in Crime

If you have high blood pressure, health problems other than heart disease may be lying in wait. Watch for these accomplices, even after hypertension has been cuffed.

Diabetes: Blood pressure and blood sugar often move in lockstep, because excess glucose damages your arterial walls, causing them to narrow. Have your fasting blood glucose checked to rule out diabetes.

Atrial fibrillation: If you lower your blood pressure but still have a large gap between the diastolic and systolic numbers, your heart may be pumping blood improperly. Atrial fibrillation (A-fib) occurs when the upper chambers of your heart aren't working in sync with the lower ones. See a cardiologist if your pressure spread is 60 points or more; that's enough to boost A-fib risk by 34 percent, according to an article in the *Journal of the American Medical Association*.

Erectile dysfunction (ED): High blood pressure and cardiovascular disease narrow the blood vessels in the penis. A urologist can determine whether a man's blood pressure is causing ED or if other factors are at work.

Kidney disease: "Hypertension might be caused by a narrowing of the renal artery that supplies blood to the kidneys," says Mark Welton, MD, an associate professor of surgery at Stanford University. And the small blood vessels inside your kidneys are vulnerable to damage from high blood pressure, boosting blood pressure even more. When high blood pressure won't respond to treatment, your doctor can do a urine test to reveal whether kidney damage is to blame.

Sleep apnea: Bedtime can be a cardiovascular nightmare if your breathing stops and starts in the middle of the night, as it does with sleep apnea. "The chronic stimulation of the nervous system caused by sleep apnea can contribute to high blood pressure," says Prediman K. Shah, MD, director of cardiology at Cedars-Sinai Medical Center in Los Angeles. The best way to identify sleep apnea is with an overnight sleep study. Find a sleep lab near you at www.sleepcenters.org.

STRESS

There was a time when stress saved your life. Blood pressure goes up in response to tension, when your body's fight-or-flight response causes adrenaline surges. But chronic stress, like the kind you experience every day at the office, can permanently increase your blood pressure set point.

Do this: Clean the house. Researchers reporting in the journal *Medicine & Science in Sports & Exercise* equipped 28 people with blood pressure monitors and asked each person to do housework to burn 150 calories a day. After 2 days, their blood pressure levels fell an average of 13 points. Daily chores lower blood pressure and not only because of the exercise. Having a clean house may reduce psychological stress, according to the study authors.

Not that: Slack off on relaxation. "Most people don't have acupuncture or perform relaxation techniques regularly enough for a lasting effect," says Dr. Shah. Reduce the chances you'll skip a de-stress session by choosing a tension reliever that's convenient and can be scheduled in advance. One option? Make a standing weekly appointment with a masseuse near your office.

A study by researchers at the University of South Florida revealed that people who received three 10-minute massages a week experienced an 18-point drop in their systolic blood pressure and an 8-point drop in their diastolic blood pressure.

YOUR GENES

Thanks to their DNA, some people can do everything right and still have high blood pressure. If your numbers are more than 20 to 30 points out of range or if your blood pressure doesn't budge with exercise and diet changes, you may need a pharmaceutical solution, says Dr. Elefteriades.

Do this: Pop more than one pill. "Many patients need additional medications to see a benefit," says Dr. Elefteriades. In fact, a new study by researchers at Trinity College in Dublin reveals that people who took a low dose of four different blood pressure drugs watched their readings drop 19 points. The combination, which included a calcium channel blocker, a beta-blocker, a diuretic, and an angiotensin-converting enzyme (ACE) inhibitor, outperformed each of the drugs on its own by as many as 10 points.

Not that: Pop painkillers for headaches. Lay off acetaminophen, ibuprofen, and other over-the-counter pain relievers if you have high blood pressure in your genes. A study published in the *Archives of Internal Medicine* found that people who regularly take painkillers have a 38 percent higher risk of developing high blood pressure.

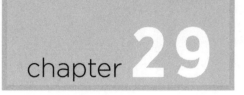
THE FRONTLINES OF THE WAR ON CANCER

Prevention's progress report on the habits, tests, and treatments that are saving lives—plus the facts you need for staying healthy

A s if being diagnosed with diabetes isn't enough, the condition sets you up for a number of other diseases as well. Researchers have found that diabetes is a risk factor for cancer. Worse, it is also associated with increased cancer mortality rates.

It's been more than 35 years since President Richard Nixon declared war on cancer. In that time, the budget of the National Cancer Institute has exploded from $500 million to nearly $5 billion, and generations of Americans have changed their lifestyles to shore up their defenses. So what do we have to show for all that money, time, and effort?

Progress—a lot of it. Yes, cancer remains a major killer of men and women. Yet treatments are more effective, tests are more precise and better able to identify disease in time to cure it, and researchers are discovering more ways to prevent wayward cells from turning into cancer in the first place. To explain why cancer is on the run, *Prevention* went to the experts. They offer hard-won insights from each of the three cancer fronts—prevention, detection, and treatment—that can make a difference in your life now.

Read about new diagnostic tests, cutting-edge treatments, and controversies in testing at www.prevention.com/cancer.

THE BATTLE FOR PREVENTION

No matter how effective cancer treatment becomes, it's clearly always better to prevent the disease. Investigators have long gathered clues about how cancer starts and how to block it, but only recently has research started to yield the details that add up to solid, effective help. Get your best shot at a cancer-free life with the following proven strategies.

Aim for a Healthy Weight

Up to 20 percent of deaths from cancer are due to people being overweight or obese.

What's new: It's now clear that being even moderately overweight can increase your cancer risk. According to Marji McCullough, ScD, RD, strategic director of nutritional epidemiology of the American Cancer Society (ACS), women who gain 11 to 22 pounds after age 18 boost their risk of breast cancer by about 15 percent.

Get Off the Couch

For decades, public health organizations have preached 30 minutes of moderate activity most days of the week to keep your heart (and the rest of your body) healthy.

What's new: Exercise cuts cancer risk, too, but getting a little extra helps even more. Go for a heart-thumping 45- to 60-minute workout 5 days a week, says Tim E. Byers, MD, MPH, professor, preventive medicine and biometrics, University of Colorado at Denver and Health Sciences Center. In a new study from UCLA, women who got sweaty for more than 5 hours per week had a 20 percent lower risk of invasive breast cancer than women who exercised 30 minutes or less weekly. Even women who start working out after menopause cut their breast cancer risk by 10 percent. "We never thought exercise would turn out to be such a key cancer fighter," says Len Lichtenfeld, MD, of the ACS.

Kick Butt

Giving up cigarettes staves off lung cancer and reduces your risk whenever you quit. Ten years after quitting, your risk of developing lung cancer is about half that of someone who's continued smoking.

What's new: That's not the only cancer payoff from quitting: The Centers for Disease Control and Prevention (CDC) estimates that at least 30 percent of all cancer deaths are due to smoking. Tobacco raises the risk of cancers of the mouth, nasal passages, larynx, throat, esophagus, stomach, liver, pancreas, kidney, bladder, and cervix.

Pile on Fruits and Veggies

Eating plenty of fresh produce reduces your chances of developing a number of cancers and precancerous conditions.

What's new: The protection is even greater than previously realized, according to studies. Research from Brigham and Women's Hospital in Boston found that women who ate five or more servings of fruit per day were 40 percent less likely than women who consumed one or fewer to develop colon polyps that can turn into cancer. And scientists at the National Cancer Institute reported that you can get a small but significant reduction in risk of head and neck cancers (6 percent) by adding just one more serving of produce a day.

Limit Hormones

Millions of women abandoned hormone therapy (HT) 5 years ago when the Women's Health Initiative reported that it increased the risk of breast cancer.

What's new: A dramatic decline in breast cancer rates confirms that the HT-cancer connection is a strong one, say researchers at Kaiser Permanente Center for Health in Portland, Oregon. The most recent stats show that breast cancer rates have dropped nearly 7 percent, falling in lockstep with the number of women on HT. Doctors now recommend that women use HT only if menopausal symptoms are making life uncomfortable, take the smallest effective dose, and stop as soon as possible.

The Supplements That Fight Cancer

The best cancer-fighting nutrients come from vitamins and minerals in food, but most of us don't get enough of them. A supplement can offer protection—just don't take more than the amounts recommended here.

Vitamin D: Studies suggest that getting enough vitamin D may cut a woman's risk of breast cancer by as much as 50 percent. People who combine vitamin D with calcium can cut the danger of developing other kinds of cancer by up to 60 percent when compared with those who take only calcium.

How much to take: 1,000 International Units (IU) a day, say experts, who call the current adequate intake level, 200 to 400 IU, woefully low.

Calcium: In a study from the ACS, people who took a calcium supplement were 30 percent less likely to develop colon cancer than those who didn't.

How much to take: 1,000 milligrams a day if you're age 50 or younger; 1,200 if older.

Folic acid: Studies have found that folic acid may reduce the risk of breast cancer by 45 percent. Some studies also link adequate folic acid with a decreased risk of colon cancer. What's more, a glass or two of wine a day raises breast cancer risk by 30 percent, but enough folic acid wipes that out.

How much to take: A multivitamin provides the necessary 400 micrograms a day.

THE INTELLIGENCE OF DETECTION

If you want to know how cancer screening can pay off, look at cervical cancer. The death rate from the disease has dropped more than 70 percent since the Pap test was introduced in the 1950s. Mortality rates for several other cancers could also drop at a considerably greater rate than we see today simply by getting people to show up for a test, experts say. If all cancers were detected at stage I or II, says Carolyn D. Runowicz, MD, director of the Carole and Ray Neag Comprehensive Cancer Center at the University of Connecticut Health Center, current therapies could cure almost every case. Says Robert A. Smith, PhD, director of cancer screening of the ACS: "Presently, nothing in our armamentarium is more effective than finding a localized tumor—before it has spread."

Comprehensive cancer screening starts in earnest at age 40. That's when women should begin scheduling an annual mammogram in addition to the Pap test they're already getting. Your first colonoscopy should come at age 50. And if you have a family history or risk factors, you may need more tests, as well. But talk with your doctor: Some exciting new exams may hold special promise for you. Here, the who, what, and why of the hot, new tests.

HPV (plus Pap) Test

A check for the human papillomavirus (HPV) strains that cause cervical cancer

Get it if: You want the most accurate way to detect cancer. When combined with a Pap test, an HPV test every 3 years is better than a Pap test alone every year, experts say. Also get an HPV test if you're under age 30 and a Pap test has shown worrisome changes. It can help determine if you need treatment.

Breast MRI

A scan that uses intense magnetic fields to produce detailed 3D pictures of the breast

Get it if: You have a mutation in the breast cancer genes (breast cancer 1, early-onset [BRCA 1] or breast cancer 2, susceptibility protein [BRCA2]). A study found that magnetic resonance imaging (MRI) picked up 77 percent of cancers in these women, compared

The Test to Skip

Computer-aided detection (CAD) technology was supposed to catch more breast cancers. The technology uses a computer to identify suspicious spots on a mammogram before it's read by a radiologist. But a recent University of California, Davis, study found that CAD didn't catch any more tumors than standard mammography, and the number of biopsies jumped by 20 percent, almost all of them unnecessary. Most women are better off sticking to the standard exam, but ask your doc if you'll benefit from a breast MRI or digital mammogram.

with 36 percent detected by mammography. (But in women at average risk, more than 50 percent of the alarms it raises prove not to be cancer.)

Digital Mammogram

X-ray images of the breast that are digitized and put on computer, where they can be enhanced to help doctors detect abnormalities

Get it if: You're under 50 or if your doc says you have dense breast tissue. A 2005 study showed that compared with standard mammography, the test found 15 percent more cancers in women under age 50 and 11 percent more in women with dense breasts—although it provided no advantage for other women.

Spiral CT

A painless x-ray procedure in which an imaging machine rotates around the body and rapidly takes 100-plus pictures of the lungs, revealing nodules too small to be seen on a conventional x-ray

Get it if: You're over age 50 and smoked at least half a pack of cigarettes a day for 20 years or more. When scientists at Cornell University scanned 27,400 ex-smokers, they found cancer in 484—85 percent of them at an early stage. (Lung cancer is usually caught much later, when the disease is notoriously difficult to treat.) The researchers believe that treatment then affords a 92 percent chance of surviving for at least 10 years. But be aware: Studies haven't yet shown whether they're right, and the scan can prompt unnecessary invasive tests and procedures.

CA-125 Blood Test Plus Vaginal Ultrasound

A CA-125 blood test measures levels of the protein that rises when ovarian cancer is present (although an increase can also be caused by other ills). Transvaginal ultrasound uses sound waves to create images of the pelvic organs. In the past, the combined test has been so-so at best; it's sent many women for surgery who turned out not to have cancer. But in a recent University of Alabama at Birmingham study, refinements in the cutoffs used to prompt a biopsy led to much greater accuracy: One out of five women flagged had ovarian cancer.

Ovarian Cancer: Is Your Doctor Symptom Savvy?

Ovarian cancer has long been called a "silent killer," spreading through a woman's body before causing any warning signs. Many patients, however, say they complained about symptoms, only to be dismissed by their doctors. Now these complaints—bloating, pelvic pain, urinary symptoms, and difficulty eating—have been recognized by major medical groups, which urge docs to take note and follow up with further exams, such as a CA-125 blood test and a vaginal ultrasound. Most women with the symptoms won't turn out to have cancer, but the alert means that those who do have the disease may be diagnosed at a treatable stage. "We're getting better at distinguishing ovarian cancer symptoms from those we all have occasionally," says Barbara Goff, MD, professor and director of gynecologic oncology at the University of Washington. "It's important that women pay attention. With ovarian cancer, time is of the essence."

Get it if: You have a family history of ovarian cancer—or if you know you have a BRCA gene mutation, which raises the risk for ovarian as well as breast cancer.

THE FRONTLINES OF TREATMENT

For so long, many people feared cancer more than other illnesses because the diagnosis often meant death. But advances in treatment are changing that. "We can turn this disease into a chronic disorder—something you've got, but you can go to work, have a life, and be happy," says David G. Nathan, MD, president emeritus of the Dana-Farber Cancer Institute in Boston.

Some of the most prevalent types of cancer are turning out to be the most curable. A case in point: breast cancer. Fifty years ago, there was a single drug to treat it. Now there are more than 15, so if one drug stops working for a patient, she can find help from another. Even patients with advanced cancer now often live strikingly normal lives. Here are the most exciting breakthrough treatments.

Surgery That's Almost Bloodless

Surgeons don't always need to cut out a tumor now. They may freeze it (cryotherapy) or heat it with radio waves (radio frequency ablation) instead. Both require only a small incision or insertion of a probe through the skin—and cause little pain and few complications.

Fighting Cancer from Within

Scientists are using the body's own immune system to seek out and destroy malignant growths, just as if they were invading bacteria. Experimental cancer "vaccines"—used for treatment, not prevention—have proved promising for non-Hodgkin's lymphoma, melanoma, and certain types of lung cancer and are being tested in larger studies.

Tailoring Treatment to a Tumor's Genes

One dilemma in breast cancer treatment: Many women with early-stage disease would do fine without chemo, but doctors haven't been able to identify them—so lots of women have had the treatment unnecessarily. Now, a tool called Oncotype DX can test 21 tumor genes and predict whether a woman's cancer will recur if she skips the toxic drugs. (Another, MammaPrint, which tests 70 genes, was approved in 2007.) The payoff: Many women can safely take a pass. And at the University of Texas M.D. Anderson Cancer Center, doctors examine proteins on the surface of lung cancer tumors before deciding which drug therapies a patient should get. "Tumor tissue patterns tell us who is most likely to benefit from which treatments," says Roy S. Herbst, MD, PhD, chief of the section of thoracic medical oncology at the University of Texas M. D. Anderson Cancer Center.

"Smart" Drugs That Aim Carefully

Traditional chemotherapy is like a carpet bombing: It kills cancer cells and healthy cells alike. New targeted therapies home in on cancer cells but preserve healthy ones. Herceptin, for a kind of breast cancer, slashes the danger of recurrence by 52 percent. Gleevec, which targets a type of leukemia and a rare form of stomach cancer, has transformed fatal diseases into survivable ones. Doctors can choose among nearly a dozen targeted therapies.

Less-Punishing Chemo

Chemotherapy isn't the devastating rite of passage it used to be. "These days, it's rare for patients to get sick to their stomach," says David G. Nathan, MD, president emeritus of the Dana-Farber Cancer Institute in Boston, thanks to new antinausea drugs. Other medications boost white blood cells, helping patients sidestep the dangerous infections that used to accompany chemotherapy, so doctors can give anticancer drugs with fewer worries about side effects.

CANCER-PROOF YOUR BODY WITH EIGHT STEALTH STRATEGIES

The average mouse doesn't care much about skin cancer. Outside of Disney cartoons, you won't see one slathering on sunscreen before heading out to dodge cats and search for cheese. But Gary Stoner, PhD, a professor emeritus of hematology and oncology at the Ohio State University Medical Center, does care about cancer. That's why he spends his days in a lab, feeding rodents polyphenols from seaweed and learning how to shrink skin cancer–like tumors. He's a mouse's best friend. Maybe yours, too.

Stoner is just one of many researchers working to bring new weapons to the cancer battle. Some researchers study humans to take a fresh look at existing theories. Others, like Stoner, are testing tactics so bold that, so far, their only subjects have tails and whiskers.

But all these approaches (seaweed included) have one very positive thing in common: They're just plain good for you and bad for cancer cells. Here are eight strategies that just may turn the Big C into the Big See-Ya-Later. (Or, better yet, See-Ya-Never.)

Drink Pomegranate Juice

Some say this luscious, lusty red fruit is Eve's original apple, but what the pomegranate truly banishes is cancer risk. The fruit's deep red juice contains polyphenols, isoflavones, and ellagic acid, elements that researchers believe make up a potent anticancer combo. Pomegranates have been shown to delay the growth of prostate cancer in mice, and they stabilize prostate-specific antigen (PSA) levels in men who've been treated for prostate cancer. And now, University of Wisconsin at Madison researchers have learned that pomegranates may also inhibit lung cancer growth. If you currently smoke, have smoked in the past, or hang around in smoky places, the juice of the fruit could bolster your defenses.

Use it: The mice in the Wisconsin study received the human equivalent of 16 ounces of juice per day, so quaff accordingly.

Eat Blueberries

Got pterostilbene? Rutgers University researchers say this compound—which is found in blueberries—has colon cancer–fighting properties. When rats with colon cancer were fed a diet supplemented with pterostilbene, they had 57 percent fewer precancerous lesions after 8 weeks than rats not given the compound.

Eat blueberries, and you'll also benefit from a big dose of vitamin C (14 milligrams per cup). In a study of 42,340 people, New England Research Institute scientists discovered that men with the highest dietary vitamin C intake (as opposed to supplements) were 50 percent less likely to develop premalignant oral lesions than men with the lowest intake.

Use it: "About two servings daily is the human equivalent of what we fed the rats," says Bandaru Reddy, MD, PhD, a chemical-biology professor at Rutgers. Load up at breakfast: A cup and a half of blueberries over cereal, plus 8 ounces of juice and half a grapefruit (for extra vitamin C), will do the trick. If that's too much to stomach at dawn, spread it out over the course of the day.

Relax a Little

Anxiety won't only make you soil your shorts. Purdue University researchers tracked 1,600 men over 12 years and found that half of those with increasing levels of worry died during the study period. Talk about flunking the exam. Only 20 percent of the optimists died before the 12-year study was completed.

More anxiety-producing news: Thirty-four percent of the neurotic men died from some type of cancer. How neurotic are we talking? "Think of the biggest worrier you know—someone who stresses out over everything," says psychologist Daniel Mroczek, PhD, who conducted the study. "That man is probably above the 95th percentile in neuroticism.

Then think of the most cool, calm, collected man you know. He's probably below the 5th percentile."

Use it: To develop that critical, casual Jeff Spicoli vibe, learn to slow down your fast times: "The more time you spend in the present moment, the more relaxed you'll be, because most mental anguish occurs over stuff that's already happened or that may or may not happen in the future," says Claire Wheeler, MD, PhD, the author of *10 Simple Solutions to Stress.* "For the most part, right now is pretty damn good. If you practice being present while shaving, for example, eventually you'll also be more present when eating, making love, and working."

Pop Selenium

Selenium has long been thought of as a cancer fighter, but you can have too much of a good thing, says David J. Waters, PhD, DVM, director of the Gerald P. Murphy Cancer Foundation, in West Lafayette, Indiana. A study of almost 1,000 men, published in the *Journal of the National Cancer Institute,* found that when those with the lowest initial levels of selenium in their bodies received a daily supplement over a 4½-year period, they cut their prostate cancer risk by an impressive 92 percent. But men who started out with high selenium levels were rewarded with an 88 percent increase in total cancer risk when they took the supplements. Moral: It pays to get your selenium level right.

Use it: Selenium in the body is measured through toenail clippings. Send yours to the Murphy Foundation, and for less than $100 (price varies by state), they'll ship them to a lab and then inform you of your level 2 weeks later. If yours is out of range, the foundation will explain how to adjust your intake of Brazil nuts, tuna, meats, grains, and selenium supplements. Learn more at www.seleniumhealthtest.com.

Order Sushi

As mentioned, Stoner is using seaweed to fight the Big C. When he fed the polyphenols from brown seaweed to mice that had been bombarded with ultraviolet (UV) rays, their incidence of skin tumors dropped 60 percent, and the polyphenols shrank existing tumors by 43 percent. Better still, the doses that produced these effects were the equivalent of only

1 or 2 tablespoons in a human being. "Seaweed is low in calories and fat, yet it provides heart-helping fiber, bone-building calcium, and iron," says nutrition consultant Molly Morgan, RD, CDN, owner of Creative Nutrition Solutions, in Vestal, New York. "Dried, roasted seaweed sheets used in making sushi also provide vitamins A and C."

Use it: "Eat more sushi rolls," says Stoner. "It's not quite the same seaweed, but it has some of the same compounds." As a bonus, sushi itself is a great muscle food. A typical spicy tuna roll has only 290 calories but packs 24 grams of protein. Also, look for a Korean-made, seaweed-fortified drink called EntroPower (www.entropower.com), which should be hitting US health food stores soon.

Spend More Time Outside

Scientists have viewed vitamin D as a potent cancer fighter for decades, but there's never been a gold-standard trial—until now. A Creighton University study published in the *American Journal of Clinical Nutrition* found that women who supplemented their diets with 1,000 IU of vitamin D every day had a 60 to 77 percent lower incidence of cancer over a 4-year period than did women taking a placebo. "I don't think the effect is limited to women," says Joan Lappe, PhD, the lead study author. "Vitamin D is necessary for the best functioning of the immune system; it causes early death of cancer cells."

Use it: Nature intended us to make vitamin D from the sun, but depending on where you live, the time of year, and how much of an agoraphobe you are, you may not reach the optimal level of 80 nanomoles per liter of blood that way. A blood test can give you a baseline. From there, Lappe recommends supplementing with 1,100 to 2,000 IU of vitamin D in a stand-alone pill every day. Vitamin D is also in sardines, salmon, shiitake mushrooms, and reindeer meat.

Clear Your Air

Secondhand smoke may be even worse for you than we thought. A recent *American Journal of Public Health* study reveals that nonsmokers working in smoky places had three times the amount of NNK, a carcinogen, in their urine than nonsmoking workers in smoke-free environments had. And their levels of NNK rose 6 percent for every hour worked.

"There is no safe level of exposure to secondhand smoke, and the greater the exposure, the higher the risk," says the study's lead author, Michael Stark, PhD, principal investigator for the Multnomah County Health Department in Portland, Oregon.

Use it: Nine states have banned smoking in all workplaces, bars, and restaurants: Arizona, Delaware, Hawaii, Massachusetts, New York, New Jersey, Ohio, Rhode Island, and Washington. So change locations, change professions, or change the laws. As you sip your pomegranate juice, sign up with Americans for Nonsmokers' Rights at www.no-smoke.org.

Invest a Little Sweat Equity

Study after study has pointed to the cancer-beating power of exercise. Now research from Norway has found that even a tiny dose of exercise has big benefits. A study of 29,110 men published recently in the *International Journal of Cancer* shows that men who exercised just once a week had a 30 percent lower risk of metastatic prostate cancer than did men who didn't work out at all. Increasing the frequency, duration, and intensity of the exercise correlated with a further, gradual reduction in risk.

Use it: Just one bout of weekend warriorism—a company softball game, pickup basketball, racquetball with your crusty uncle—might qualify you for inclusion in the cancer-free 30 percent.

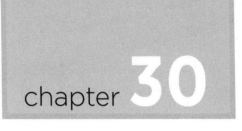

chapter 30

THE SUGAR-SKIN CONNECTION

Learn why uncontrolled blood sugar can cause wrinkles—and five steps to help ensure that it won't

People with diabetes know the ravaging effects of sugar all too well. It can affect your nerves, circulation, vision, and much more. But did you know that years of out-of-control blood sugar can also make your skin show early signs of aging?

At blame is a natural process that's known as glycation, in which the sugar in your bloodstream attaches to proteins to form harmful new molecules called advanced glycation end products (or, appropriately, AGEs for short). The more sugar you eat, the more AGEs you develop.

"As AGEs accumulate, they damage adjacent proteins in a domino-like fashion," explains Fredric Brandt, MD, a dermatologist and author of *10 Minutes/10 Years*. Most vulnerable to damage are collagen and elastin—the protein fibers that keep skin firm and elastic. Once damaged, they turn from springy and elastic to dry and brittle, leading to wrinkles and sagging. These effects start at about age 35 and rapidly increase after that, according to a study published in the *British Journal of Dermatology*.

"Depending on how well their disease is controlled, diabetics can have up to 50 times the number of AGEs in their skin as those who don't have diabetes," says Karyn Grossman, MD, a dermatologist and chief of the division of dermatology at St. John's Hospital in Santa Monica, California.

Besides damaging collagen, a high-sugar diet also affects what type of collagen you have, which is another factor in how resistant skin is to wrinkling, says Dr. Brandt. The most abundant collagens in the skin are types I, II, and III, with type III being the most stable and longest lasting. Glycation transforms type III collagen into type I, which is more fragile. "When that happens, the skin looks and feels less supple," says Dr. Brandt. The final blow: AGEs deactivate your body's natural antioxidant enzymes, leaving you more vulnerable to sun damage, which is still the main cause of skin aging.

But here's the good news about sugar-damaged skin: It's never too late to turn back the clock. One way is to build new collagen with products that contain retinoids. Look for retinol in over-the-counter serums and lotions or prescription creams such as Renova, Avage, and Differin. Then, to keep this new collagen supple, you can prevent AGEs from forming by taking steps to minimize the damage that sugar causes to your skin. Here are five steps to eat right and keep your skin looking its youngest.

CUT BACK ON THE SWEET STUFF

It's not easy to eliminate sugar completely. During digestion, even whole grains, fruits, and vegetables turn to glucose, which is the type of sugar that fuels glycation. But limiting added sugar can help. Here are some guidelines.

Count carbs wisely. When you read nutrition facts labels, remember that the "grams of total carbohydrates" includes not only sugar but also complex carbs and fiber. By the same token, don't judge a food by its sugars alone: Some foods that appear high in sugar are also rich in nutrients (say, milk and fruit). And foods with no added sugars (such as some cereals and grains) can still be high in carbs, which can boost blood sugar if eaten in excess. Talk to your doctor if you're not sure how many grams of carbohydrates to aim for in a day.

Watch for hidden sugar in food. Many prepared foods contain hefty amounts of sugar, but it's hidden under aliases—including barley malt, corn syrup, dextrose, fruit juice concentrate, maltose, maple syrup, molasses, and turbinado—on ingredient panels. The key is determining how many teaspoons of sugar each serving contains. Doing this is easy: Check the nutrition label for sugars, which are listed in grams under total carbohydrates. Divide the grams of sugar by 4 to convert it to teaspoons. (Each teaspoon of sugar is equal to 4 grams.) For example, if sugars are listed as 12 grams, you're getting 3 teaspoons of sugar per serving.

Avoid high-fructose corn syrup (HFCS). This type of sweetener, which is made by changing the sugar in cornstarch to fructose (another form of sugar), is believed to produce more AGEs than other types. Because HFCS extends the shelf life of foods and is sweeter and cheaper than other sugars, it's a popular ingredient in soda, fruit-flavored drinks, and packaged foods such as breads, crackers, and other snacks. You can spot it in ingredient lists on nutrition labels.

SUPPLEMENT YOUR DIET WITH B VITAMINS

Aim for at least 1 milligram of B_1 and B_6 a day. In a number of published studies, these vitamins proved to be potent AGE inhibitors, says David J. Goldberg, MD, a New York City–based dermatologist and clinical professor of dermatology at Mount Sinai School of Medicine. Vitamins B_1 and B_6 are plentiful in food, but taking a multivitamin—most of which deliver at least 1 milligram of both Bs—ensures that you're getting the daily value of 1.1 milligrams for B_1 and 1.3 milligrams for B_6 (1.5 milligrams after age 50).

WEAR BROAD-SPECTRUM SPF 30 SUNSCREEN EVERY DAY

Yes, even in cold weather. Significantly more AGEs occur in sun-exposed skin than in protected skin, according to the *British Journal of Dermatology* study.

The number of "appearance" years women say they would erase to boost their confidence: 10 years

EMPLOY AN INSIDE-OUT APPROACH TO ANTIOXIDANTS

These free-radical fighters help keep sugar from attaching to proteins, so replenishing their supply is important. First, focus on eating more antioxidant-rich fruits, nuts, and vegetables, such as cranberries, walnuts, and red bell peppers. Second, apply topical antioxidants such as vitamins C and E. "It seems to be the best way to ensure that they reach the dermal layer of skin, where collagen and elastin are located," says Dr. Goldberg.

USE NEW INGREDIENTS THAT PROTECT SKIN FROM SUGAR

A growing number of products contain compounds such as aminoguanidine and alistin, which have been shown to block the formation of AGEs.

"Aminoguanidine attaches to molecules that start the glycation process and prevents them from binding to collagen and elastin," explains Dr. Grossman. "Alistin acts as a decoy, so it gets damaged instead of the proteins in your skin." In a study on Prescriptives Anti-AGE Advanced Protection Lotion SPF 25 ($60; www.prescriptives.com), which contains both ingredients, skin treated with the product had 21 percent fewer AGEs after 8 weeks than untreated skin. Now that's sweet!

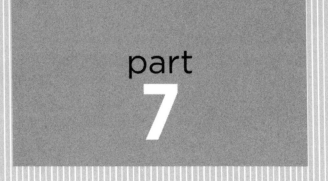

part
7

DIABETES COOKBOOK

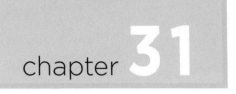

chapter 31

THE RECIPES

ere are more than 100 of the very best of this year's *Prevention* recipes, specifically selected for people with diabetes. Besides tasting great, they're healthy to boot.

When selecting these recipes, we divided the FDA's daily value for calories— 2,000—by four meals a day to get 500 calories per meal. Then, because according to the National Heart, Lung, and Blood Institute, you should get no more than 60 percent of your calories from carbs, we kept each entrée's carbohydrates below 75 grams, each snack less than 30 grams, and each side dish less than 25 grams. But if you eat more than one dish per meal, take that into account. And be sure to coordinate your medicine with your meals.

BREAKFASTS

APPETIZERS AND SNACKS

SALADS

SOUPS

VEGETARIAN AND SIDE DISHES

CHICKEN AND TURKEY MAIN DISHES

BEEF, PORK, LAMB, AND MORE MAIN DISHES

FISH AND SEAFOOD MAIN DISHES

BREAKFASTS

Egg-and-Cheese Sandwich

1	egg
2	slices whole wheat bread
2	slices reduced-sodium deli ham (We used Healthy Choice.)
1	slice low-fat Cheddar cheese
1	slice tomato
2	romaine lettuce leaves

1. Lightly coat a nonstick skillet with cooking spray and add the egg. (Break the yolk if you want to.)

2. While the egg is frying, toast the bread and layer the ham, cheese, tomato, and romaine on one slice, with the lettuce on the bottom. Top with the cooked egg and the remaining slice of bread.

Makes 1 serving

Per serving: 305 cal, 25 g pro, 29 g carb, 10 g fat, 3 g sat fat, 223 mg chol, 5 g fiber, 776 mg sodium

Exchanges: 1½ starch, 1 fat, 2 meat, ½ vegetables, 1 very lean meat

Breakfast Burrito

$^1/_4$	cup diced lean lower-sodium ham
1	large (8") whole wheat tortilla
1	large egg + 4 large egg whites, beaten
$^1/_4$	cup fresh cilantro
$^1/_4$	cup shredded low-fat Cheddar cheese
2	tablespoons salsa

1. In a nonstick skillet coated with cooking spray, sauté the ham over medium-high heat, until the surface just starts to brown. Place the cooked ham in the tortilla.

2. Then add more cooking spray to the skillet and scramble the eggs together with the cilantro. Add the eggs to the tortilla, top with the cheese and salsa, and fold.

Makes 1 serving

Per serving: 374 cal, 37 g pro, 24 g carb, 11 g fat, 3 g sat fat, 232 mg chol, 3 g fiber, 805 mg sodium

Exchanges: 1 starch, 1 fat, 2 meat, 0 vegetable, 3 very lean meat

Breakfast Pita

See photo insert.

4	white mushrooms, sliced	3	egg whites
1	tablespoon chopped onion	$^1/_2$	small tomato, seeded and chopped
1	tablespoon chopped red bell pepper	3	tablespoons water or 1 percent milk
	Pinch of freshly ground black pepper	1	whole wheat pita, halved and toasted
1	egg	$^1/_2$	avocado, sliced

1. Coat a skillet with cooking spray and place over medium heat. Add the mushrooms, onion, bell pepper, and black pepper. Cook for 3 to 4 minutes.

2. Meanwhile, in a bowl, combine the egg, egg whites, tomato, and water or milk. Whisk together until frothy. Pour the egg mixture into the skillet. Cook, stirring, for 3 to 4 minutes, or until the eggs are firm. Fill each pita with half the eggs, and top with the avocado.

Makes 1 serving

Per serving: 437 cal, 27 g pro, 41 g carb, 20 g fat, 3 g sat fat, 212 mg chol, 11 g fiber, 563 mg sodium

Exchanges: ½ fruit, 3 fat, 1 meat, 1 vegetable, 1½ very lean meat

Grilled Sausage with the Works

½	tablespoon extra virgin olive oil		2	cloves garlic, minced
6	ounces precooked chicken sausage		½	teaspoon red-pepper flakes
1	red or yellow bell pepper, sliced		1	tablespoon balsamic vinegar
1	medium red onion, sliced			Salt
1	large portobello mushroom cap, sliced			Freshly ground black pepper
			1	cup soft polenta, prepared according to package directions

1. Heat a grill pan or cast-iron skillet over medium-high heat and add the oil.

2. When the oil begins to smoke, add the sausage, pepper, onion, and mushroom. Cook for 3 to 4 minutes, moving the vegetables with a pair of tongs or a spatula so they cook evenly. Add the garlic, pepper flakes, and vinegar and cook for another 3 to 4 minutes, until the vegetables and sausage are browned and the vinegar has been absorbed. Season to taste with salt and black pepper.

3. Divide the polenta onto two plates. Top with the sausage and vegetables.

Makes 2 servings

Per serving: 299 cal, 20 g pro, 26 g carb, 13 g fat, 6 g sat fat, 60 mg chol, 3 g fiber, 327 mg sodium

Exchanges: ½ starch, 1 fat, 2½ meat, 2 vegetable

Avocado Toast

2	teaspoons honey mustard
2	slices whole-grain bread, toasted
$\frac{1}{2}$	avocado, peeled and sliced
$\frac{1}{2}$	tomato, thinly sliced
1	teaspoon extra virgin olive oil
4	fresh basil leaves, chopped
$1\frac{1}{2}$	teaspoons ground flaxseed
	Salt
	Freshly ground black pepper

1. Spread the honey mustard on the toast slices. Layer on the avocado and tomato. Drizzle with the oil.

2. Top with the basil and flaxseed, and season with salt and pepper to taste.

Makes 1 serving

Per serving: 364 cal, 9 g pro, 41 g carb, 21 g fat, 3 g sat fat, 0 mg chol, 12 g fiber, 481 mg sodium

Exchanges: 1½ starch, ½ fruit, 3½ fat, ½ vegetable

Variations: Add a few thin slices of cucumber, a pinch of Parmesan cheese, or fresh baby spinach leaves.

Toast with Tuna

1	can (6 ounces) solid white tuna		2	teaspoons balsamic vinegar
2	tablespoons dried cranberries, roughly chopped			Salt
				Freshly ground black pepper
$\frac{1}{4}$	yellow onion, minced		2	pieces whole-grain bread, toasted
1	tablespoon mayonnaise			

1. In a medium bowl, mix together the tuna, cranberries, onion, mayonnaise, and vinegar. Season to taste with salt and pepper.

2. Place one piece of toast on each of two plates, and divide the tuna between them.

Makes 2 servings

Per serving: 229 cal, 22 g pro, 23 g carb, 6 g fat, 1 g sat fat, 38 mg chol, 6 g fiber, 262 mg sodium

Exchanges: ½ starch, ½ fruit, ½ fat, ½ vegetable

Whole Wheat French Toast with Pumpkin Butter

See photo insert.

1	teaspoon unsalted butter
1	egg + 1 egg white, beaten
2	slices whole wheat bread
1	tablespoon pumpkin butter (available at specialty and gourmet stores)

1. In a frying pan, melt the butter over medium heat.

2. In a bowl, beat together the egg and egg white. Dip the bread into the mixture, coating thoroughly.

3. Add the bread to the pan and cook both sides until golden brown. Serve with the pumpkin butter.

Makes 1 serving

Per serving: 283 cal, 17 g pro, 30 g carb, 11 g fat, 4 g sat fat, 222 mg chol, 4 g fiber, 393 mg sodium

Exchanges: 1½ starch, ½ other carbohydrate, 1½ fat, 1 meat, ½ very lean meat

French Toast with Whipped Fruit Topping

1½	cups low-fat, low-sodium cottage cheese
	Splenda
1	cup blueberries
2	eggs + 2 egg whites, beaten
¾	cup low-fat milk
1	teaspoon ground cinnamon
½	teaspoon vanilla extract
6	slices whole-grain bread

1. In a bowl, using an electric mixer on high speed, blend the cottage cheese, Splenda to taste, and ½ cup of the blueberries on high for 30 seconds, or until smooth and creamy. Set aside.

2. In a large bowl, mix together the eggs and egg whites, milk, cinnamon, and vanilla. Soak the bread one slice at a time until it's saturated with liquid, then cook it over medium-high heat on a nonstick skillet coated with cooking spray until lightly browned on both sides. Serve with the whipped fruit topping and put the remaining blueberries on top.

Makes 2 servings

Per serving: 493 cal, 42 g pro, 58 g carb, 11 g fat, 4 g sat fat, 223 mg chol, 7 g fiber, 569 mg sodium

Exchanges: 2½ starch, ½ milk, ½ fruit, 1 fat, 1 meat, 3½ very lean meat

Almond-Pecan Waffles

1	cup almond flour
¼	cup finely chopped pecans
1	teaspoon baking powder
4	ounces regular cream cheese, softened
6	eggs
¼	cup heavy cream
¼	cup sugar-free maple syrup

1. Preheat a waffle iron.

2. Meanwhile, in a small bowl, combine the almond flour, pecans, and baking powder.

3. In another bowl, whisk the cream cheese and two of the eggs until smooth. Add the remaining eggs one at a time, and whisk thoroughly after each. Mix in the cream, then stir in the dry ingredients.

4. Spoon about ⅓ cup of the batter onto the hot waffle iron and cook about 3 minutes, or until golden brown. Top with the syrup.

Makes about six 7-inch waffles

Note: You can make almond flour by chopping slivered almonds in a food processor, or you can purchase it preground at www.bobsredmill.com.

Per serving: 318 cal, 12 g pro, 8 g carb, 28 g fat, 9 g sat fat, 246 mg chol, 3 g fiber, 233 mg sodium

Exchanges: 5 fat, 1 meat

Cottage-Cheese Pancakes

1	cup cottage cheese
2	eggs
$\frac{1}{2}$	stick butter, melted
$\frac{1}{2}$	cup milk
$\frac{3}{4}$	cup whole wheat flour
1	tablespoon baking powder
1	tablespoon sugar
1	teaspoon salt
$\frac{1}{2}$	teaspoon nutmeg (optional)

1. In a large bowl, stir together the cheese, eggs, butter, and milk. Add the flour, baking powder, sugar, salt, and nutmeg (if desired), and blend lightly until just mixed.

2. Coat a griddle with cooking spray and place over medium heat. Put a large scoop of the batter on the griddle, and use the back of a spoon to spread it out evenly. The pancake is ready to flip when you begin to see small air bubbles form, about 3 to 4 minutes. Flip and cook for another minute or 2.

Makes about 12 4-inch pancakes

Per pancake: 96 cal, 5 g pro, 8 g carb, 5 g fat, 3 g sat fat, 47 mg chol, 1 g fiber, 436 mg sodium

Exchanges: $\frac{1}{2}$ starch, 1 fat, $\frac{1}{2}$ very lean meat

Yogranola

1   cup low-fat plain yogurt

½   cup low-fat granola

Put the yogurt in a bowl and stir in the granola.

Makes 1 serving

Note: If desired, sweeten the plain yogurt with Splenda.

Per serving: 363 cal, 17 g pro, 61 g carb, 7 g fat, 3 g sat fat, 15 mg chol, 3 g fiber, 306 mg sodium

Exchanges: 2½ starch, 1½ milk, ½ fat

Mocha Custard

2   cups low-fat sugar-free chocolate milk

2   cups strong coffee (regular or decaf)

3   eggs, beaten
            Pinch of salt
            Splenda

1. In a saucepan, combine the milk, coffee, eggs, salt, and Splenda to taste. Whisk to mix well. Gently cook over medium heat, stirring constantly, until the mixture begins to thicken and lightly coats the back of a spoon.

2. Remove from the heat, pour into a covered pitcher, and cool quickly by placing the pitcher into an ice-water bath until it's half submerged. Serve chilled.

Makes 4 servings

Per serving: 122 cal, 10 g pro, 9 g carb, 5 g fat, 2 g sat fat, 166 mg chol, 0 g fiber, 185 mg sodium

Exchanges: ½ other carbohydrate, ½ fat, ½ meat

APPETIZERS AND SNACKS

Pitas with Tzatziki

2	cups low-fat plain Greek-style yogurt (We used Fage 2 percent.)
1	cup peeled, grated cucumber, spun dry in salad spinner
4	cloves garlic, grated
1	teaspoon freshly squeezed lemon juice
3/4	teaspoon kosher salt
1/8	teaspoon ground red pepper
3	large whole wheat pitas (6"–7" diameter)
1	tablespoon extra virgin olive oil

1. In a medium bowl, make tzatziki by mixing together the yogurt, cucumber, garlic, lemon juice, salt, and pepper. Cover and chill for 1 hour.

2. Brush both sides of the pitas lightly with the oil. In a large skillet over medium heat, warm the pitas in batches, 3 to 4 minutes per side, until golden and puffed. Cut the pitas into triangles. Serve the pitas with the tzatziki.

Makes 6 servings

Per serving: 155 cal, 9 g pro, 22 g carb, 5 g fat, 2 g sat fat, 3 mg chol, 5 g fiber, 433 mg sodium

Exchanges: 1 starch, 1/2 fat

Tuna Salad on Celery Sticks

1	can (6 ounces) low-sodium chunk white tuna (packed in water), rinsed and drained
1	tablespoon balsamic vinegar
$\frac{1}{4}$	cup finely chopped onion
$\frac{1}{4}$	cup finely chopped apple
2	tablespoons fat-free plain yogurt
	Dash of ground black pepper
14	ribs celery, rinsed and ends trimmed

1. Put the tuna in a small bowl and break it apart with a fork. Add the vinegar, onion, apple, yogurt, and pepper. Mix well.

2. Spoon an equal amount of tuna salad into the gutter of each celery rib. Cover with plastic wrap and refrigerate until you're ready to eat.

Makes 7 servings

Per serving: 58 cal, 8 g pro, 7 g carb, 1 g fat, 0 g sat fat, 11 mg chol, 2 g fiber, 118 mg sodium

Exchanges: 1 vegetable

Peach-Mango Salsa with Pita Chips

See photo insert.

1	cup chopped grape tomatoes (about 20)			Juice of 1 lime
1	small mango, peeled, seeded, and chopped (about 3/4 cup)		1	tablespoon red wine vinegar
3/4	cup chopped Grilled Peaches (2–3 halves)(See recipe on page 297.)		1	tablespoon sugar or honey

1   cup chopped grape tomatoes
       (about 20)

1   small mango, peeled, seeded, and
       chopped (about ³⁄₄ cup)

³⁄₄   cup chopped Grilled Peaches (2–3
       halves)(See recipe on page 297.)

¹⁄₂   medium red bell pepper, finely
       chopped (about ¹⁄₃ cup)

¹⁄₂   small onion, finely chopped (about
       ¹⁄₄ cup)

¹⁄₄   cup fresh cilantro leaves, chopped

1   jalapeño chile, seeded and finely
       chopped (Wear plastic gloves when
       handling.)

Juice of 1 lime

1   tablespoon red wine vinegar

1   tablespoon sugar or honey

1   tablespoon orange juice

¹⁄₈   teaspoon salt

3   large whole wheat pitas (6"–7"
       diameter), each cut into 8 wedges
       and peeled apart

1   teaspoon salt-free garlic and herb
       seasoning blend (We used Mrs.
       Dash.)

1.   Preheat the oven to 350°F.

2.   In a medium bowl, combine the tomatoes, mango, peaches, bell pepper, onion, cilantro, and chile.

3.   In a small bowl, whisk together the lime juice, vinegar, sugar or honey, orange juice, and salt. Add to the tomato mixture and stir well. Chill, covered, at least 1 hour to blend flavors.

4.   Place the pita wedges on a large baking sheet and coat lightly with cooking spray. Sprinkle the wedges with the seasoning blend. Bake for 5 to 6 minutes, or until the edges just start to brown. Cool and serve with the salsa.

Makes 6 servings

Per serving: 144 cal, 4 g pro, 30 g carb, 2 g fat, 0 g sat fat, 0 mg chol, 4 g fiber, 223 mg sodium

Exchanges: 1 starch, ¹⁄₂ fruit, ¹⁄₂ vegetable

One-Dish Baba Ghannouj

2	cups finely chopped Grilled Eggplant (about 4 large slices) (See recipe on page 300.)
2	tablespoons finely chopped fresh cilantro
1	tablespoon white wine vinegar
1	tablespoon tahini paste
2	cloves garlic, smashed to a paste with a pinch of kosher salt
2	teaspoons extra virgin olive oil
$\frac{1}{2}$	teaspoon ground cumin
$\frac{1}{2}$	teaspoon ground coriander
$\frac{1}{4}$	teaspoon red-pepper flakes
$\frac{1}{4}$	teaspoon kosher salt

In a medium bowl, mix together all ingredients. Let stand at room temperature 30 minutes or longer to blend flavors.

Makes 4 servings

Note: Serve as a dip with pita crisps and bell peppers, or pair with soft goat cheese as a spread for crostini.

Per serving: 106 cal, 2 g pro, 8 g carb, 8 g fat, 1 g sat fat, 0 mg chol, 4 g fiber, 365 mg sodium

Exchanges: 1½ fat, 1 vegetable

Crudités with Romesco Sauce

3	large red bell peppers		4	carrots, trimmed and cut into 2"–3" strips
3	tablespoons extra virgin olive oil		1	large or 2 small cucumbers, cut into 2"–3" strips
2	tablespoons sliced almonds		1	bulb fennel, trimmed and cut into 2"–3" strips
2	cloves garlic, smashed			
1	plum tomato, quartered		1/2	pound yellow wax beans, trimmed
1	slice multigrain bread, cubed		1/2	pound green beans, trimmed
1	tablespoon red wine vinegar			
1	teaspoon paprika			
3/4	teaspoon salt			
1/4	teaspoon freshly ground black pepper			

1. Preheat the broiler with the rack about 4" from the heat.

2. Place the 3 bell peppers on a baking sheet and broil, turning every 3 minutes, until the skins are blistered and charred, for 12 to 15 minutes. Transfer the peppers to a medium bowl, cover with plastic wrap, and let steam for 10 minutes. Peel, and discard the stems, seeds, and ribs.

3. In a small skillet, combine the oil, almonds, and garlic over medium heat. Cook, stirring often, until the almonds and garlic are lightly golden, about 4 to 5 minutes. Remove from the heat.

4. Put the roasted peppers and tomato in a blender and puree. Add the oil mixture and bread, and puree. Pour in the vinegar, paprika, salt, and black pepper, and puree. Transfer to a serving bowl and chill the sauce for 20 minutes, or until ready to serve.

5. Arrange the carrots, cucumbers, fennel, and beans on a platter. Serve with the romesco sauce.

Makes 8 servings

Per serving: 125 cal, 3 g pro, 16 g carb, 7 g fat, 1 g sat fat, 0 mg chol, 5 g fiber, 279 mg sodium

Exchanges: 1 fat, 2½ vegetable

Sweet Potato–Coconut Fritters

2	6-ounce sweet potatoes, peeled and cut into chunks
1	teaspoon water
1	egg yolk
1	tablespoon cornmeal
1	teaspoon jarred minced garlic in oil
1	teaspoon minced fresh ginger
$\frac{1}{2}$	teaspoon baking powder
$\frac{1}{8}$	teaspoon salt
3	tablespoons flaked coconut

1. Place the sweet potatoes on a microwavable plate with the water. Cover with microwave-safe plastic wrap, and microwave on high until soft, about 6 minutes. Let stand for 3 minutes. Mash with a fork.

2. Preheat the oven to 350°F. Coat a nonstick baking sheet with cooking spray.

3. In a food processor with a steel blade, pulse the potatoes, egg yolk, cornmeal, garlic, ginger, baking powder, and salt. Pulse about 6 times, scraping down the sides of the container as needed, until a coarse puree forms. Drop the batter onto the pan in 24 equal dollops. Top each with some of the coconut, pressing gently to adhere. Bake until the coconut starts to brown, about 15 minutes. Serve warm or at room temperature.

Makes 12 servings

Per serving: 31 calories, 1 g pro, 5 g carbs, 1 g fat, 0.5 g sat fat, 17 mg chol, 1 g fiber, 52 mg sodium

Exchanges: $\frac{1}{2}$ starch

Crunchy Parmesan Herb Chicken Tenders

1	pound skinless, boneless chicken tenders, cut into 24 equal pieces
1/4	cup whole wheat pastry flour
1/3	cup plain panko crispy bread crumbs (We used Progresso.)
1/2	cup grated Parmesan cheese
1/2	teaspoon jarred minced garlic in oil
1/2	teaspoon minced fresh rosemary
1/8	teaspoon salt
1/8	teaspoon freshly ground black pepper
1	large egg white
1	tablespoon water

1. Preheat the oven to 425°F. Coat a baking sheet with olive oil cooking spray.

2. Lightly coat the chicken with the flour.

3. On a plate, combine the panko, Parmesan, garlic, rosemary, salt, and pepper.

4. In a bowl, beat the egg and add the water.

5. Dip one chicken piece at a time into the egg white, then into the crumbs, shaking off the excess after each dip, and place on the pan. Lightly spritz the breaded pieces with the olive oil. Bake for 7 minutes. Flip and bake for 8 more minutes until the tenders are crispy and the juices run clear.

Makes 12 servings

Per serving: 67 cal, 11 g pro, 3 g carb, 2 g fat, 0.6 g sat fat, 25 mg chol, 0 g fiber, 101 mg sodium

Exchanges: 1 very lean meat

Beef and Asparagus Rolls with Lemon-Horseradish Cream

½	pound asparagus stalks
¾	cup 1 percent small-curd cottage cheese
3	tablespoons horseradish
2	teaspoons grated lemon zest
1	pound sliced delicatessen roast beef, halved

1. Preheat the oven to 400°F.

2. Place the asparagus on a baking sheet and spritz with vegetable oil cooking spray. Roll the stalks to coat with the oil. Roast for about 7 minutes, or until the skin blisters. Remove and cool.

3. Meanwhile, in a food processor with a metal blade, combine the cottage cheese, horseradish, and lemon zest. Pulse about 12 times, until smooth.

4. Lay the roast beef on a work surface. Spread 1 teaspoon of the horseradish mixture on each slice. Cut the asparagus stalks in half and center both pieces of each stalk across each beef slice. Fold a small flap of meat over the non-tip end of each stalk, and then roll into cornucopias with the asparagus tips peeking out the ends. Arrange on a serving platter.

Makes 16 servings

Per serving: 47 cal, 7 g pro, 1 g carb, 1 g fat, 0.4 g sat fat, 16 mg chol, 0 g fiber, 210 mg sodium

Exchanges: 1 very lean meat

Pesto-Stuffed Baby 'Bello Mushrooms

24	baby portobello mushrooms (about 1 pound)
$\frac{1}{2}$	cup part-skim ricotta cheese
2	tablespoons refrigerated pesto (We used Buitoni.)
2	teaspoons whole wheat pastry flour
2	tablespoons grated Pecorino Romano cheese
1	tablespoon dry breadcrumbs
	Grape tomato for garnish, slivered (optional)

1. Preheat the oven to 400°F. Coat a baking sheet with cooking spray.

2. Remove the stems from the mushrooms and lay on pan, hollow side up.

3. In a bowl, mix the ricotta cheese, pesto, and flour until smooth. Spoon a dollop of the mixture into each cap, smoothing with the back of a spoon.

4. In another bowl, combine the Pecorino Romano cheese and breadcrumbs, and sprinkle on top of the pesto mixture. Press lightly to adhere. Bake for about 15 minutes, or until hot and browned. Serve warm or at room temperature, garnished with a sliver of grape tomato, if desired.

Makes 12 servings

Per serving: 49 cal, 3 g pro, 3 g carb, 3 g fat, 1 g sat fat, 5 mg chol, 1 g fiber, 59 mg sodium

Exchanges: ½ fat, ½ meat, ½ vegetable

Cajun Meatballs

1	pound pork tenderloin, cut into small chunks
2	tablespoons minced fresh parsley
2	teaspoons jarred minced garlic in oil
2	teaspoons Cajun seasoning (We used Spice Islands World Flavors Louisiana Style.)
$\frac{1}{4}$	teaspoon salt

1. Preheat the oven to 375°F. Coat a large baking pan with olive oil cooking spray.

2. In a food processor with a steel blade, pulse the pork with the parsley, garlic, seasoning, and salt about 16 times, or until evenly ground. With clean hands, roll the mixture into 32 meatballs. Place on the prepared pan and spritz lightly with olive oil cooking spray. Bake for about 10 minutes, or until the meat is no longer pink and the juices run clear.

Makes 16 servings

Per serving: 39 cal, 6 g pro, 0 g carb, 1 g fat, 0 g sat fat, 18 mg chol, 0 g fiber, 118 mg sodium

Exchanges: 1 very lean meat

Candylike Almonds

20	raw almonds
1	teaspoon ground cinnamon
1	packet sugar substitute (We used Splenda.)

1. Preheat the oven to 350°F.

2. Spread the almonds in a single layer on a nonstick baking sheet and roast for 7 to 10 minutes.

3. Transfer the almonds to a small bowl and spritz several times with zero-calorie butter or cooking spray. Sprinkle with the cinnamon and the sugar substitute, and toss until well coated.

4. Cool for 5 minutes.

Makes 2 servings

Per serving: 75 cal, 3 g pro, 4 g carb, 6 g fat, 1 g sat fat, 0 mg chol, 2 g fiber, 7 mg sodium

Exchanges: 1 fat, ½ meat, ½ very lean meat

Spicy Roasted Nuts

2	cups unsalted almonds
2	cups unsalted pecan halves
1	cup unsalted walnut halves
$\frac{1}{4}$	teaspoon ground red pepper
2	teaspoons dried rosemary
2	teaspoons dried oregano
2	teaspoons paprika (smoked or regular)
2	teaspoons ground black pepper
$\frac{1}{2}$	teaspoon salt
2	tablespoons extra virgin olive oil

1. Preheat the oven to 300°F.

2. In a bowl, combine the almonds, pecans, walnuts, red pepper, rosemary, oregano, paprika, black pepper, and salt and toss to coat the nuts evenly. Add the oil a tablespoon at a time, tossing well after each addition. Spread the nuts on a baking sheet in an even layer. Bake for 30 minutes, stirring occasionally, or until golden brown.

3. Set the mix aside to cool before storing in a plastic container or zipper-lock bag.

Makes 20 servings

Per serving: 240 cal, 6 g pro, 6 g carb, 24 g fat, 2 g sat fat, 0 mg chol, 4 g fiber, 59 mg sodium

Exchanges: ½ starch, 4 fat, ½ meat, ½ very lean meat

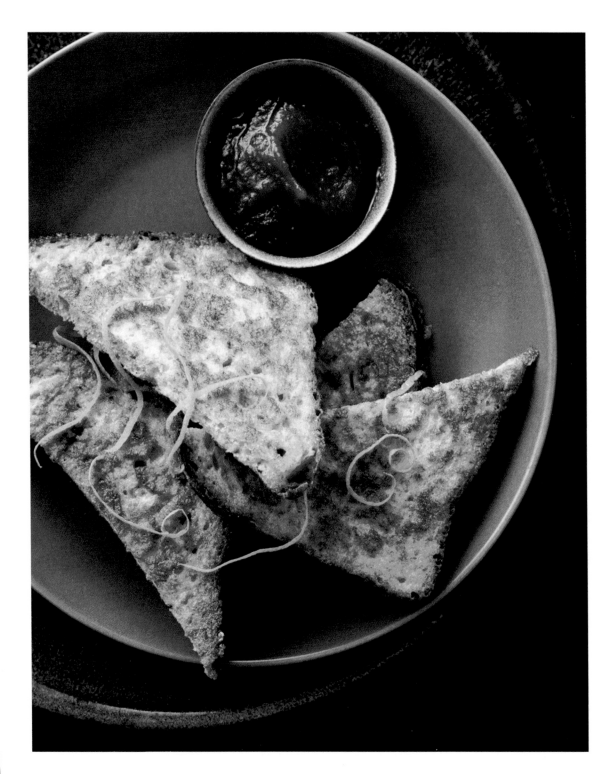

Whole Wheat French Toast with Pumpkin Butter
Recipe on page 263

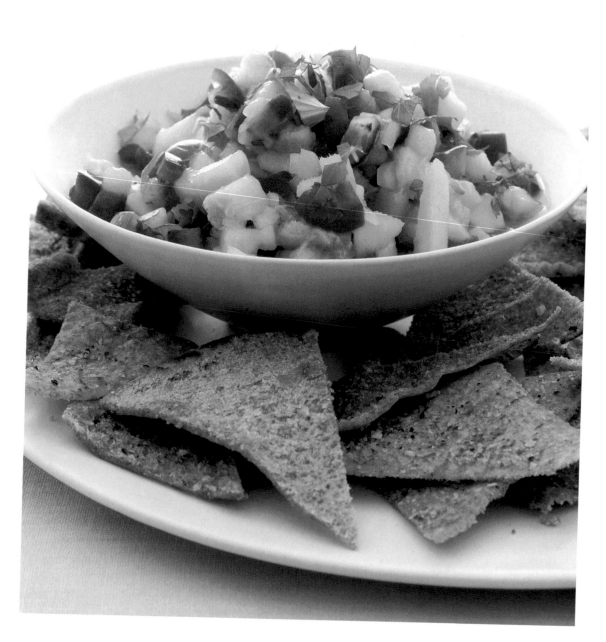

Peach-Mango Salsa with Pita Chips
Recipe on page 270

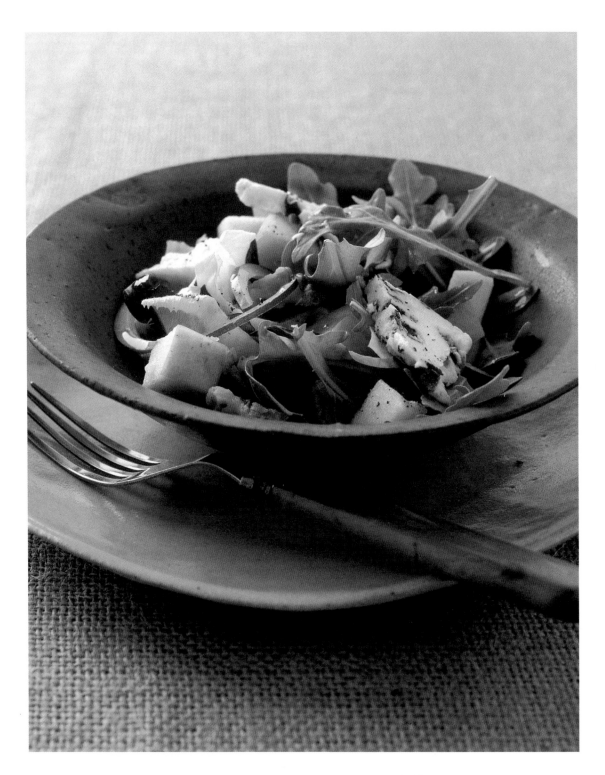

Apple Salad with Radicchio, Roquefort, and Walnuts
Recipe on page 280

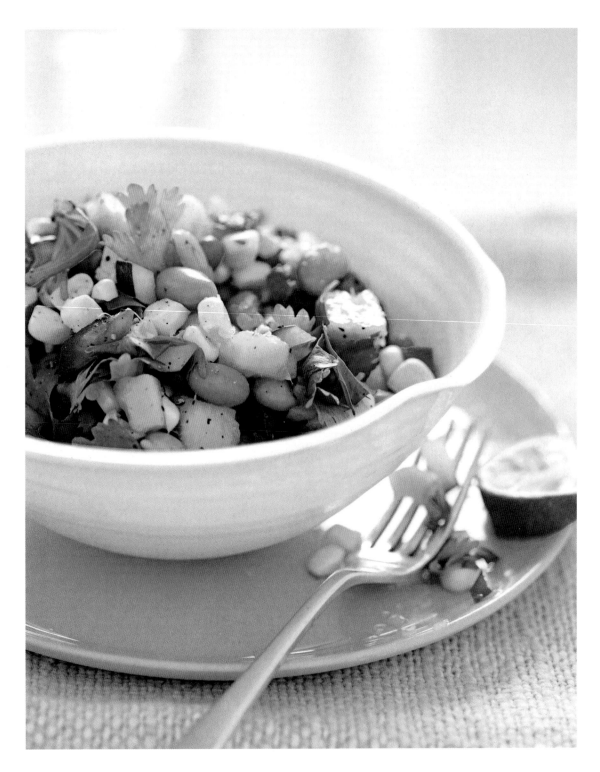

Corn, Mango, and Edamame Salad
Recipe on page 282

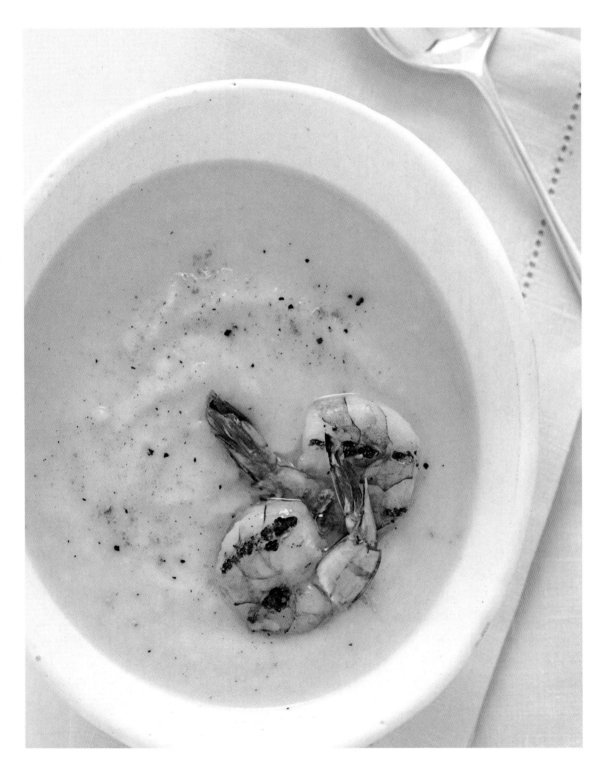

Cauliflower Soup with Grilled Shrimp
Recipe on page 288

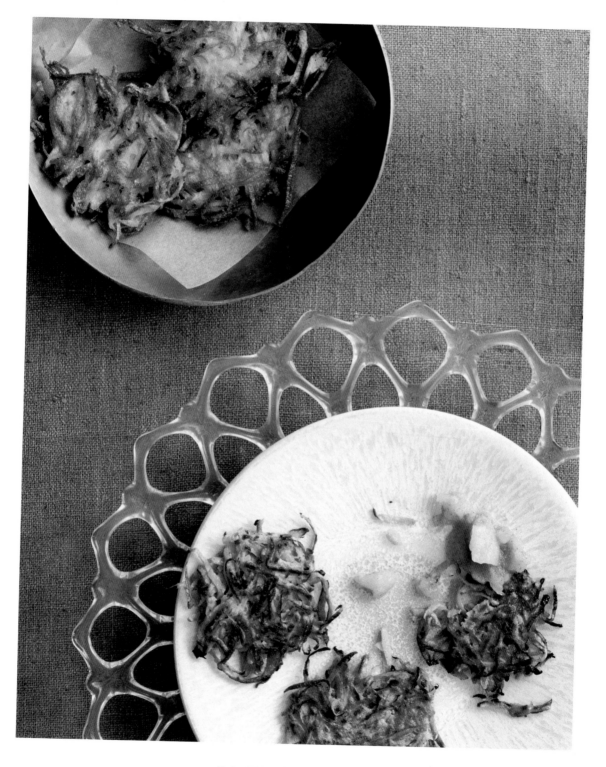

Baked Sweet Potato Latkes
Recipe on page 298

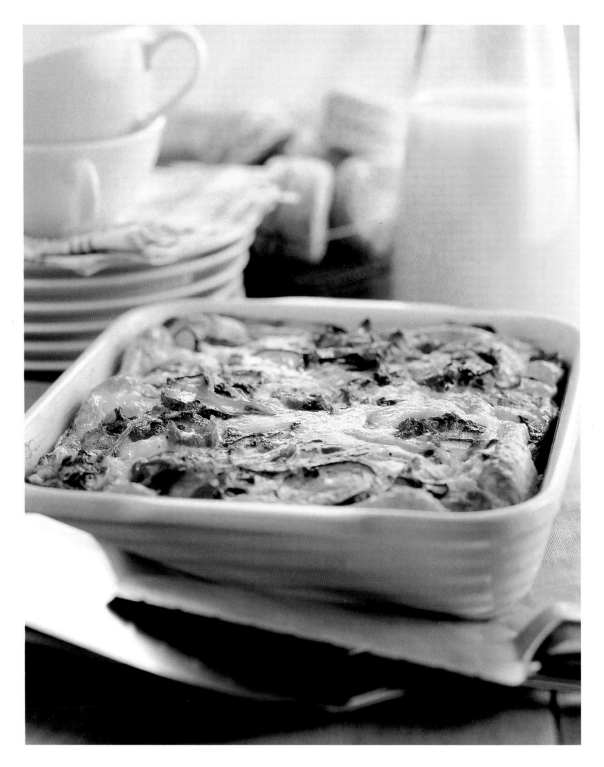

Zucchini Casserole
Recipe on page 303

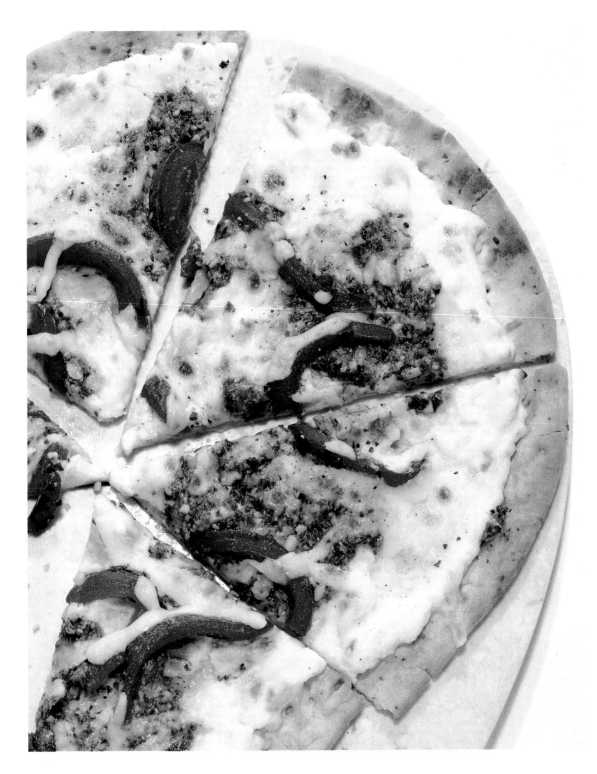

Red Pepper Pesto Pizza
Recipe on page 309

SALADS

Simple Blue Cheese Salad

2⅓	cups mixed greens
¼	cup canned kidney beans, drained
1	tablespoon chopped onion
1	tablespoon crumbled blue cheese
	Pinch of freshly ground black pepper
1	tablespoon red wine
1	teaspoon olive oil

Put the greens into a bowl. Add the beans, onion, cheese, pepper, wine, and oil. Toss to combine.

Makes 1 serving

Per serving: 183 cal, 9 g pro, 19 g carb, 8 g fat, 2 g sat fat, 6 mg chol, 9 g fiber, 151 mg sodium

Exchanges: 1 starch, 1 fat, ½ meat, 1 vegetable

Greek Salad

5	cups mixed greens
2	roma tomatoes, chopped
½	cup chopped cucumber
2	tablespoons shredded mozzarella cheese
	Pinch of freshly ground black pepper
2	tablespoons balsamic vinegar
2	teaspoons olive oil

In a mixing bowl, toss together the greens, tomatoes, cucumber, cheese, pepper, vinegar, and oil.

Makes 2 servings

Per serving: 113 cal, 5 g pro, 10 g carb, 7 g fat, 2 g sat fat, 6 mg chol, 4 g fiber, 86 mg sodium

Exchanges: 1 fat, 1½ vegetable

Baby Spinach Salad with Goat Cheese and Toasted Pistachios

2	tablespoons balsamic vinegar
1	tablespoon extra virgin olive oil
	Dash of salt
	Dash of freshly ground black pepper

4	cups loosely packed baby spinach
2	ounces crumbled goat cheese
2	tablespoons shelled pistachio nuts, toasted

1. Place the vinegar into a medium bowl. Whisk in the oil. Season with the salt and pepper.

2. In a medium bowl, toss the spinach in the vinaigrette, using tongs to coat the spinach evenly. Divide the spinach between two plates and top with the cheese and nuts.

Makes 2 servings

Per serving: 241 cal, 9 g pro, 11 g carb, 19 g fat, 7 g sat fat, 22 mg chol, 3 g fiber, 305 mg sodium

Exchanges: 3 fat, 1 meat, 1 vegetable

Apple Salad with Radicchio, Roquefort, and Walnuts

See photo insert.

2	large Golden Delicious apples, cored and chopped
1	small head radicchio, chopped
2	Belgian endives, chopped
1	cup chopped arugula
$\frac{1}{8}$	cup thinly sliced red onion
2	tablespoons extra virgin olive oil
2	tablespoons lemon juice
2	tablespoons apple cider vinegar

1	clove garlic, minced
$\frac{1}{4}$	teaspoon kosher salt
$\frac{1}{8}$	teaspoon freshly ground black pepper
2	ounces Roquefort cheese, crumbled (about $\frac{1}{3}$ cup)
2	tablespoons chopped walnuts, toasted

1. In a large bowl, mix together the apples, radicchio, endive, arugula, and onion.

2. In a small bowl, whisk together the oil, lemon juice, vinegar, garlic, salt, and pepper. Toss with the apple mixture, cheese, and walnuts.

Makes 4 servings

Per serving: 207 cal, 5 g pro, 19 g carb, 14 g fat, 4 g sat fat, 13 mg chol, 4 g fiber, 384 mg sodium

Exchanges: 1 fruit, 2½ fat. ½ meat, 1 vegetable

Village Salad with Feta

1	large English cucumber, peeled and sliced ¼" thick (3 cups)
3	medium tomatoes, halved and sliced ¼" thick (3 cups)
1	large onion, halved and sliced ¼" thick (1 cup)
2	ounces feta cheese, sliced, or ½ cup feta cheese crumbles
6	kalamata olives, pitted and halved lengthwise
2	tablespoons extra virgin olive oil
½	teaspoon kosher salt
½	teaspoon dried oregano
⅛	teaspoon ground red pepper

1. Alternate slices of the cucumber and tomato around the rim of a large platter, spiraling inward. Scatter the onion on top. Layer on the feta and scatter the olives over the top.

2. Drizzle all over with the oil. Sprinkle with the salt, oregano, and pepper.

Makes 6 servings

Per serving: 109 cal, 3 g pro, 7 g carb, 8 g fat, 2 g sat fat, 8 mg chol, 2 g fiber, 333 mg sodium

Exchanges: 1½ fat, 1 vegetable

Corn, Mango, and Edamame Salad

See photo insert.

2	cups frozen shelled edamame		2	tablespoons chopped fresh cilantro
1½	cups fresh corn kernels (from 2 large ears)		1	tablespoon extra virgin olive oil
1½	cups mango cubes (about 1 medium mango)		1	tablespoon freshly squeezed lime juice
1	cup chopped tomato (about 1 large)		¾	teaspoon salt
½	cup chopped red onion (about 1 small)		¼	teaspoon freshly ground black pepper

1. Prepare the edamame per the package directions. Drain and rinse under cold water.

2. Transfer the edamame to a large bowl. Stir in the corn, mango, tomato, onion, cilantro, oil, lime juice, salt, and pepper. Toss well.

Makes 6 servings

Per serving: 159 cal, 9 g pro, 22 g carb, 5 g fat, 0.4 g sat fat, 0 mg chol, 6 g fiber, 303 mg sodium

Exchanges: 1 starch, ½ fruit, ½ fat, ½ vegetable, 1 very lean meat

Quinoa Salad

¼	cup uncooked quinoa		1	tablespoon extra virgin olive oil
¼	cup chopped parsley			Juice of ½ lemon or lime
¼	cup finely chopped onion			Ground black pepper
½	cucumber, peeled and chopped		1	leaf romaine lettuce (optional)
2	plum tomatoes, diced			

1. Cook the quinoa according to the package directions. Allow it to cool.

2. In a bowl, toss all the ingredients. Serve on a bed of romaine, if using.

Makes 2 servings

Per serving: 174 cal, 4 g pro, 22 g carb, 9 g fat, 1 g sat fat, 0 mg chol, 3 g fiber, 14 mg sodium

Exchanges: 1 starch, 1½ fat, 1 vegetable

Eggplant and Chickpea Salad with Cherry Tomatoes

4	cups cubed (½") Grilled Eggplant (about 8 large slices) (See recipe on page 300.)
1	can (16 ounces) no-salt-added chickpeas, rinsed and drained (1½ cups)
1	cup cherry tomatoes, cut crosswise into ¼"-thick slices
1	tablespoon finely chopped fresh parsley
2	tablespoons red wine vinegar
2	tablespoons extra virgin olive oil
1	tablespoon freshly squeezed lemon juice
2	cloves garlic, minced
½	teaspoon freshly grated lemon zest
¼	teaspoon freshly ground black pepper

1. In a large bowl, toss the eggplant, chickpeas, tomatoes, and parsley.

2. In a small bowl, whisk together the vinegar, oil, lemon juice, garlic, lemon zest, and pepper. Pour over the salad and toss gently to coat. Let stand at least 20 minutes at room temperature to blend flavors. (Chill if not serving within 2 hours.)

Makes 8 servings

Per serving: 203 cal, 5 g pro, 23 g carb, 11 g fat, 2 g sat fat, 0 mg chol, 10 g fiber, 497 mg sodium

Exchanges: 2 fat, 2½ vegetable, ½ very lean meat

Avocado Black Bean Salad

2	cups chopped romaine lettuce hearts
1	medium avocado, chopped into bite-size pieces
1	medium tomato, chopped into bite-size pieces
1/2	cup canned black beans, rinsed and drained
2	tablespoons diced green onion
1	tablespoon diced fresh cilantro
1	tablespoon olive oil
2	teaspoons lime juice
1/4	teaspoon lime zest
1/4	teaspoon salt
1/2	teaspoon ground black pepper

1. In a large bowl, toss together the lettuce, avocado, tomato, beans, green onion, and cilantro.

2. In a small bowl, stir together the oil, lime juice, lime zest, salt, and pepper. Pour over the salad, and toss well to coat.

Makes 2 servings

Per serving: 261 cal, 7 g pro, 21 g carb, 22 g fat, 2 g sat fat, 0 mg chol, 8 g fiber, 530 mg sodium

Exchanges: 1/2 starch, 4 fat, 1 vegetable

Israeli Couscous Salad

2	cups water
1	cup Israeli (or pearl) couscous
1	tablespoon rice wine vinegar
1	tablespoon extra virgin olive oil
1	tablespoon orange juice
1	teaspoon white miso paste
8	ounces steamed large shrimp
2	clementines or small oranges, peeled and sectioned
1	tablespoon finely chopped fresh cilantro
$\frac{1}{4}$	teaspoon kosher salt
$\frac{1}{8}$	teaspoon freshly ground black pepper
$\frac{1}{2}$	avocado, peeled and cubed

1. In a medium saucepan, bring the water to a boil. Add the couscous and boil for 10 minutes. Drain and rinse with cold water. Set aside.

2. In a large bowl, whisk together the vinegar, oil, orange juice, and miso paste. Add the couscous, shrimp, clementines, and cilantro, and toss well. Sprinkle with the salt and pepper, add the avocado, and toss gently.

Makes 6 servings

Per serving: 186 cal, 11 g pro, 23 g carb, 5 g fat, 1 g sat fat, 74 mg chol, 3 g fiber, 204 mg sodium

Exchanges: 1 fat, 1 starch, 1 meat

SOUPS

Southwest Bean Potage

1	tablespoon sunflower oil
2	cups chopped onion and red bell pepper
1	tablespoon garlic, minced
2	teaspoons ground cumin
$\frac{1}{2}$	teaspoon salt
1	can (15 ounces) pumpkin
1	can (15.5 ounces) unsalted pinto beans, rinsed and drained (We used Eden brand.)
4	cups fat-free reduced-sodium vegetable broth
2	cups (2 ounces) baby spinach leaves, shredded
4	teaspoons chopped roasted pumpkin seeds
4	lime wedges or a few drops sherry vinegar (optional)

1. In a pot, heat the oil over medium heat. Add the onion, pepper, garlic, cumin, and salt. Cover and sauté, stirring occasionally, until the onion is softened, about 5 minutes.

2. Add the pumpkin, pinto beans, and broth. Simmer for 10 minutes to let the flavors blend.

3. Stir in the spinach. Cook for 2 minutes to wilt. Sprinkle the seeds on each serving. Serve with the lime or a few drops of vinegar to taste, if desired.

Makes 6 servings

Note: Using bagged spinach and precut onions and peppers from the frozen-food section or salad bar of your supermarket, makes this recipe easy.

Per serving: 141 cal, 5 g pro, 24 g carb, 3 g fat, 0 g sat fat, 0 mg chol, 7 g fiber, 673 mg sodium

Exchanges: ½ starch, ½ fat, 1 vegetable, 1 very lean meat

Turkey, Barley, and Greens Soup

1	tablespoon canola oil
1	cup chopped onion
1	cup chopped carrot
8	ounces ground turkey breast
1½	teaspoons poultry seasoning
½	teaspoon ground black pepper
	Salt
¾	cup quick-cooking barley
4	cups fat-free reduced-sodium chicken broth
2	cups water
2	cups (4 ounces) mustard greens, coarsely chopped

1. In a pot, heat the oil over medium heat. Add the onion and carrot. Cover and sauté, stirring occasionally, until the vegetables are lightly browned, about 5 minutes.

2. Increase the heat to high and add the turkey, poultry seasoning, pepper, and salt to taste. Sauté, breaking the turkey into small chunks, until the meat is no longer pink, about 3 minutes.

3. Add the barley. Cook, stirring, for 2 minutes. Add the broth and water. Bring to a boil.

4. Reduce the heat to simmer on medium-low and add the greens. Simmer until the barley is cooked, about 10 minutes.

Makes 6 servings

Per serving: 178 cal, 14 g pro, 25 g carb, 3 g fat, 0 g sat fat, 15 mg chol, 6 g fiber, 347 mg sodium

Exchanges: 1 starch, ½ fat, 1 vegetable, 1 very lean meat

Cauliflower Soup with Grilled Shrimp

See photo insert.

3	teaspoons olive oil, divided
1	cup chopped red onion (1 medium)
$\frac{1}{2}$	cup chopped celery
4	cups cauliflower florets (about $1\frac{1}{2}$ pounds)
$\frac{1}{2}$	teaspoon ground coriander
2	cans (14.5 ounces each) low-sodium chicken or vegetable broth
12	ounces large shrimp, peeled and deveined (8–12 shrimp)
$\frac{1}{2}$	teaspoon salt, divided
$\frac{1}{4}$	teaspoon freshly ground black pepper, divided
$\frac{1}{3}$	cup fat-free evaporated milk

1. Preheat the grill to medium-high. Coat a grill rack with cooking spray.

2. In a soup pot, heat 2 teaspoons of the oil over medium heat. Add the onion and celery and cook, stirring occasionally, for 6 to 7 minutes. Stir in the cauliflower and coriander. Cook for 2 minutes. Add the broth and bring to a boil. Reduce the heat to medium-low, cover, and simmer until tender, for 20 minutes. Remove from the heat and cool for 5 minutes.

3. In a bowl, season the shrimp with $\frac{1}{4}$ teaspoon of the salt, $\frac{1}{8}$ teaspoon of the pepper, and the remaining 1 teaspoon of oil. Grill until opaque, for 2 to 3 minutes per side.

4. In a blender, puree the soup in batches. Return it to the pot. Stir in the milk and the remaining salt and pepper. Warm over medium heat until heated through, about 5 minutes. Serve with the shrimp.

Makes 4 servings

Per serving: 198 cal, 23 g pro, 17 g carb, 6 g fat, 1 g sat fat, 127 mg chol, 5 g fiber, 579 mg sodium

Exchanges: $\frac{1}{2}$ fat, 2 vegetable, $2\frac{1}{2}$ very lean meat

Potato Corn Chowder with Scallops

3	strips turkey bacon
$\frac{1}{2}$	cup chopped green onions (about 4)
1	cup chopped celery
2	cups peeled and chopped potatoes (about 2 medium)
$2\frac{1}{2}$	cups low-fat milk
1	cup bottled clam broth
$1\frac{1}{2}$	cups fresh or frozen corn kernels
$\frac{3}{4}$	pound bay scallops
3	tablespoons chopped fresh parsley, divided

1. In a 3-quart microwavable casserole dish, cook the bacon in a single layer on high for 4 to 5 minutes, or until crisp. Remove and chop. Return all but 2 tablespoons to the dish.

2. Add the green onions and celery to the dish and cook on high for 4 to 5 minutes, or until soft. Add the potatoes, milk, and broth. Cover tightly with microwave-safe plastic wrap, and cook on high for 13 to 15 minutes.

3. Add the corn and cook on high for 2 minutes. Remove $1\frac{1}{2}$ cups of the soup mixture (leave the rest in the dish) and purée in a blender or mash with a potato masher.

4. Return the puree to the dish. Add the scallops and 2 tablespoons of the parsley. Cook on high for 3 minutes, or until the scallops are opaque.

5. Ladle the soup into bowls. Crumble the reserved bacon over each serving. Top with the remaining parsley.

Makes 6 servings

Per serving: 164 cal, 17 g pro, 18 g carb, 3 g fat, 1 g sat fat, 31 mg chol, 3 g fiber, 335 mg sodium

Exchanges: $\frac{1}{2}$ starch, $\frac{1}{2}$ milk, $\frac{1}{2}$ vegetable, $1\frac{1}{2}$ very lean meat

Creamy Potato, Kale, and Leek Soup

12	ounces red potatoes, unpeeled
1	tablespoon canola oil
3	cups (6 ounces) chopped kale, tightly packed
3	cups chopped leek, white and pale-green parts (2 medium leeks)
1/2	teaspoon salt
3	cups 1 percent milk
1/4	teaspoon ground nutmeg
	Ground black pepper

1. Cut the potatoes into golf ball-size pieces and place on a microwave-safe plate. Cover with waxed paper. Cook on high, rotating occasionally, until tender, for about 6 minutes.

2. Meanwhile, in a pot, heat the oil for 1 minute over medium heat. Add the kale, leek, and salt. Stir. Cover and cook, stirring occasionally, until softened, about 5 minutes.

3. Add the milk, potatoes, and nutmeg. Reduce the heat to medium-low. With a potato masher or the back of a large spoon, smash the potatoes into small chunks. Simmer until the flavors blend, about 5 minutes. Sprinkle each serving with pepper to taste.

Makes 6 servings

Per serving: 156 cal, 7 g pro, 25 g carb, 4 g fat, 1 g sat fat, 6 mg chol, 3 g fiber, 274 mg sodium

Exchanges: 1/2 starch, 1/2 milk, 1/2 fat, 2 vegetable

Seafood Fennel Chowder

1½	tablespoons extra virgin olive oil
2	cups chopped fennel bulb + 2 tablespoons chopped fresh fennel leaves (See note.)
1	cup chopped red onion
1	tablespoon minced garlic
1	can (14 ounces) petite diced salt-free tomatoes with juice
4	cups fat-free reduced-sodium chicken broth
	Salt
⅛	teaspoon red pepper flakes
½	pound tilapia fillet, cut into large chunks
1	pouch (2.5 ounces) whole baby clams, rinsed and drained
¼	pound shrimp, peeled and deveined
4	orange wedges (optional)

1. In a pot, heat the oil over medium heat. Add the fennel bulb, onion, and garlic. Cover and sauté, stirring occasionally, until the onion browns, about 4 minutes.

2. Add the tomatoes with juice, broth, salt to taste, and pepper flakes. Bring to a boil.

3. Add the tilapia. Bring to a boil. Reduce the heat and simmer for 5 minutes.

4. Add the clams and shrimp. Simmer until the shrimp is opaque and the clams open, about 3 minutes.

5. Sprinkle with the fennel leaves. Squeeze an orange wedge over each serving, if desired.

Makes 4 servings

Note: Florence fennel (often mislabeled "anise") can be found in most supermarket produce sections.

Per serving: 214 cal, 23 g pro, 12 g carb, 8 g fat, 1 g sat fat, 86 mg chol, 3 g fiber, 677 mg sodium

Exchanges: 1 fat, 2 vegetable, 3 very lean meat

Wild Salmon Bisque

1	tablespoon canola oil
³/₄	cup finely chopped onion
¹/₂	cup bottled roasted red pepper, drained and chopped
2	teaspoons herbes de Provence
¹/₄	cup whole wheat pastry flour
¹/₄	cup cold water
5	cups 1 percent milk, divided
2	pouches (6 ounces each) wild pink salmon
¹/₄	teaspoon hot-pepper sauce
¹/₈	teaspoon salt
4	teaspoons chopped parsley

1. In a saucepan, heat the oil over medium-low heat. Add the onion, red pepper, and herbs. Sauté until the onion is softened, about 5 minutes.

2. In a bowl, whisk the flour and water until smooth. Gradually add 1 cup of the milk and whisk. Add the mixture to the saucepan with the remaining 4 cups of milk. Cook, stirring, until the mixture bubbles and thickens.

3. Add the salmon, hot-pepper sauce, and salt. Reduce the heat to low. Simmer for 5 minutes.

4. In a food processor or with a hand-held blender, process the soup into a coarse puree. Garnish with the parsley.

Makes 4 servings

Per serving: 306 cal, 29 g pro, 25 g carb, 10 g fat, 3 g sat fat, 60 mg chol, 1 g fiber, 506 mg sodium

Exchanges: ¹/₂ starch, 1¹/₂ milk, 1 fat, ¹/₂ vegetable, 2¹/₂ very lean meat

Spiced Butternut Soup with Crab

4	cups Roasted Butternut Squash (See page 302.)
3	cups low-sodium chicken broth
$\frac{1}{4}$	cup whole milk
$\frac{1}{2}$	teaspoon ground cumin
	Pinch of freshly ground nutmeg
	Dash of hot-pepper sauce
$\frac{1}{4}$	teaspoon kosher salt
$\frac{1}{8}$	teaspoon freshly ground black pepper
6	ounces cooked lump crabmeat

1. In a blender, combine the squash, broth, milk, cumin, nutmeg, and hot-pepper sauce (or use an immersion blender) and puree. Transfer to a medium saucepan.

2. Heat over medium heat for 7 minutes and season with the salt and pepper. (If the soup is too thick, add additional broth to reach the desired consistency.) Divide the soup among 4 bowls and top each with $1\frac{1}{2}$ ounces of crabmeat.

Makes 6 servings

Per serving: 148 cal, 10 g pro, 21 g carb, 4 g fat, 1 g sat fat, 29 mg chol, 3 g fiber, 368 mg sodium

Exchanges: $\frac{1}{2}$ fat, 3 vegetable, 1 very lean meat

Beef Soup with Soba Noodles

4	cups low-sodium beef broth
3	cups water
1	tablespoon low-sodium soy sauce
6	ounces frozen shaved beef sandwich steaks, cut into strips
1	teaspoon toasted sesame oil
2	ounces dried soba noodles or whole wheat spaghetti
$\frac{1}{2}$	cup slivered green onions
$\frac{1}{2}$	cup shredded carrots
$\frac{1}{2}$	cup fresh cilantro leaves
4	lime wedges
1	fresh hot red or green chile, thinly sliced, seeds removed (Wear plastic gloves when handling.)

1. Bring a pot of water to boil over high heat.

2. Meanwhile, in another pot, bring the broth, water, and soy sauce to a simmer over high heat. Add the beef and sesame oil. Reduce the heat to low.

3. Add the noodles to the first pot of boiling water. Cook, stirring, until al dente, about 4 minutes.

4. Divide the noodles into four large soup bowls. Ladle the beef and broth mixture over the noodles. Garnish with the green onions, carrots, cilantro, lime, and chile.

Makes 4 servings

Per serving: 249 cal, 14 g pro, 16 g carb, 14 g fat, 6 g sat fat, 30 mg chol, 2 g fiber, 468 mg sodium

Exchanges: $\frac{1}{2}$ starch, 2 fat, 1$\frac{1}{2}$ meat, $\frac{1}{2}$ vegetable

Ultimate Game-Day Chili

1	pound extra-lean ground beef
1	onion, diced
3	cloves garlic, crushed
2	cans (15 ounces each) kidney beans, rinsed and drained
2	cans (8 ounces each) diced tomatoes
2	cans (10.75 ounces each) chicken broth
$\frac{1}{2}$	teaspoon salt
$\frac{1}{2}$	teaspoon ground black pepper
1	teaspoon chili powder
$\frac{1}{2}$	teaspoon cumin
$\frac{1}{8}$	teaspoon red pepper
$\frac{1}{8}$	teaspoon cinnamon
1	ounce dark chocolate

1. In a nonstick skillet, brown the beef over medium-high heat. Remove it with a slotted spoon and set it aside, leaving some of the fat in the skillet. Sauté the onion and garlic in the fat until soft, about 6 minutes.

2. In a large stockpot, combine the browned beef, sautéed onion and garlic, beans, tomatoes, broth, salt, pepper, chili powder, cumin, red pepper, cinnamon, and chocolate. Simmer on low heat for 1 hour.

Makes 6 servings

Per serving: 229 cal, 24 g pro, 23 g carb, 6 g fat, 2 g sat fat, 40 mg chol, 10 g fiber, 376 mg sodium

Exchanges: ½ fat, 1 vegetable, 3 very lean meat

VEGETARIAN AND SIDE DISHES

Beer Bread

3	cups self-rising flour
2	tablespoons sugar
1	can (12 ounces) light beer, room temperature
1	egg
1	tablespoon water

1. Preheat the oven to 375°F. Coat a nonstick bread pan with cooking spray.

2. In a large bowl, mix the flour, sugar, and beer. Pour into the prepared pan. Let the dough sit until it has doubled in size, about 15 minutes.

3. In a small bowl, beat the egg with the water. Brush the top of the bread with the egg mixture. Bake 1 hour.

Makes 16 servings

Per serving: 100 cal, 3 g pro, 19 g carb, 1 g fat, 0 g sat fat, 13 mg chol, 1 g fiber, 303 mg sodium

Exchanges: 1 starch

Grilled Peaches

8   halved, pitted peaches

1   tablespoon toasted walnut oil

         Freshly ground black pepper

1. Preheat the grill to medium.

2. Brush the peaches on all sides with the oil. Place on the grill cut-side down and grill for 10 to
    12 minutes, turning once, or until heated through but still holding shape. Remove the peels, if
    desired.

3. Sprinkle with the pepper.

Makes 8 servings

Per serving: 53 cal, 1 g pro, 9 g carb, 2 g fat, 0 g sat fat, 0 mg chol, 0 mg sodium, 2 g dietary fiber

Exchanges: ½ fruit, ½ fat

Garlic-Chive Mashed Potatoes

6	baking potatoes
2	cups 1 percent milk
$^2/_3$	cup fat-free sour cream
1	teaspoon salt
1	teaspoon garlic powder
	Freshly ground black pepper
3	tablespoons freshly minced chives

1. Preheat the oven to 425°F.

2. Bake the potatoes until soft, about 1 hour, and remove from the oven.

3. Scoop out the potato flesh and mash it. Place it into a large bowl.

4. Add the milk, sour cream, salt, garlic, and black pepper to taste. Mix well and top with the chives.

Makes 10 servings

Per serving: 122 cal, 4 g pro, 25 g carb, 1 g fat, 1 g sat fat, 4 mg chol, 1 g fiber, 271 mg sodium

Exchanges: 1 starch

Baked Sweet Potato Latkes

See photo insert.

2	pounds grated sweet potatoes
1	medium onion, finely chopped
2	eggs, beaten
$^1/_4$	cup flour
$^1/_4$	teaspoon baking powder
$^1/_2$	teaspoon salt
$^1/_2$	teaspoon ground cinnamon
$^1/_4$	teaspoon ground nutmeg

1. Preheat the oven to 400°F. Coat two baking sheets with cooking spray.

2. In a large bowl, combine all ingredients. Drop by quarter-cupfuls onto the baking sheets. Flatten with a spatula.

3. Bake for 25 minutes. Flip and bake for an additional 10 minutes.

Makes 15 servings

Per serving: 87 cal, 2 g pro, 18 g carb, 0 g fat, 0 g sat fat, 28 mg chol, 2 g fiber, 115 mg sodium

Exchanges: 1 starch

Lemon Roasted Potatoes

1/4	cup water
2	tablespoons extra virgin olive oil
1	teaspoon kosher salt
1/2	teaspoon dried oregano
1/8	teaspoon freshly ground black pepper
2	pounds boiling potatoes, peeled and cut lengthwise into 1/2" wedges
2	tablespoons lemon juice

1. Preheat the oven to 425°F. Pour the water into a 12" × 9" baking dish.

2. In a large mixing bowl, whisk together the oil, salt, oregano, and pepper. Add the potatoes and toss. Pour into the baking dish.

3. Roast the potatoes for 30 minutes, turning halfway through. Drizzle the lemon juice over the top and roast 10 to 15 minutes longer, until the potatoes are browned and cooked through.

Makes 8 servings

Per serving: 130 cal, 2 g pro, 23 g carb, 4 g fat, 1 g sat fat, 0 mg chol, 2 g fiber, 246 mg sodium

Exchanges: 1½ starch, ½ fat

Grilled Eggplant

4	eggplants (1 pound each), with peel, cut lengthwise into 1"-thick slices
2	teaspoons kosher salt, divided
4	tablespoons extra virgin olive oil
$\frac{1}{4}$–$\frac{1}{2}$	teaspoon freshly ground black pepper

1. Layer several paper towels on a baking sheet. Place half of the eggplant on top in a single layer. Sprinkle with 1 teaspoon of the salt, and cover with paper towels. Arrange a second layer of eggplant, sprinkle with the remaining salt, and cover with paper towels.

2. Let the eggplant stand for 30 minutes, then rinse each piece and blot dry. (This step helps extract excess water, reducing the bitterness and preventing the eggplant from absorbing excess oil during cooking.)

3. Brush both sides of an eggplant slice with the oil to coat and transfer to a large bowl. Repeat with the remaining oil and eggplant slices. Season with the pepper.

4. Heat the grill to medium.

5. Grill the eggplant, with the cover closed, for 16 to 20 minutes, turning once, until the eggplant is browned and tender. Refrigerate the leftovers in an airtight container for a day or two.

Makes 8 servings

Per serving: 118 cal, 2 g pro, 13 g carb, 7.5 g fat, 1 g sat fat, 0 mg chol, 8 g fiber, 485 mg sodium

Exchanges: 1½ fat, 2 vegetable

Slow-Roasted Tomatoes

3	pounds firm, ripe plum tomatoes (20–24), trimmed and halved lengthwise
2	tablespoons minced garlic
2	teaspoons finely chopped fresh thyme
2	tablespoons olive oil (preferably extra virgin)
1	teaspoon kosher salt
¼	teaspoon freshly ground black pepper

1. Preheat the oven to 250°F. Line two large baking sheets with parchment paper.

2. Place the tomatoes cut-side up on the prepared baking sheets. Sprinkle garlic and thyme on each and drizzle with the oil, spreading it over the surface with your fingertips. Season with the salt and pepper and roast 4 to 5 hours, until the tomatoes are dried but still moist.

3. Refrigerate the leftovers in an airtight container for up to 1 week.

Makes 8 servings

Per serving: 71 cal, 1 g pro, 7 g carb, 4 g fat, 1 g sat fat, 0 mg chol, 2 g fiber, 248 mg sodium

Exchanges: ½ fat, 1½ vegetable

Roasted Butternut Squash

8	cups prepackaged cubed (1") butternut squash (about 4 pounds peeled, seeded, and cubed)
2	tablespoons olive oil
1	teaspoon ground cumin
1	teaspoon kosher salt
$\frac{1}{2}$	teaspoon ground allspice
$\frac{1}{2}$	teaspoon ground coriander
$\frac{1}{4}$	teaspoon freshly ground black pepper

1. Preheat the oven to 425°F.

2. In a large bowl, toss the squash with the oil.

3. In a small bowl, combine the cumin, salt, allspice, coriander, and pepper. Sprinkle the squash with the spices and toss well to evenly coat.

4. Spread the squash in a single layer on 2 baking sheets or pans and roast for 40 minutes, turning every 10 minutes.

Makes 10 servings

Per serving: 112 cal, 2 g pro, 23 g carb, 3 g fat, 0.4 g sat fat, 0 mg chol, 4 g fiber, 200 mg sodium

Exchanges: ½ fat, 3½ vegetable

Zucchini Casserole

See photo insert.

2	egg whites
1	medium zucchini
1	medium eggplant
1½	cups bread crumbs
1	teaspoon garlic powder
1	teaspoon low-sodium Italian seasoning
1	package (8 ounces) shredded, low-fat mozzarella cheese
1	jar (48 ounces) fat-free, low-sodium pasta sauce

1. In a small bowl, beat the egg whites.

2. Slice the zucchini and eggplant into ¼"-thick rounds.

3. In another small bowl, mix the bread crumbs, garlic powder, and seasoning.

4. Set aside ½ cup of the cheese.

5. Dip the sliced eggplant in the egg whites and then in the bread crumb mixture. Layer in a slow cooker, pouring ½ jar of the sauce over the top. Spread evenly and sprinkle with half of the remaining cheese. Repeat the next layer using the zucchini slices. Top with the remaining sauce and cheese.

6. Cover. Cook on low for 5 to 6 hours. Top with the reserved ½ cup of cheese before the last 15 minutes of cooking.

Makes 8 servings

Per serving: 204 cal, 15 g pro, 28 g carb, 5 g fat, 3 g sat fat, 15 mg chol, 5 g fiber, 346 mg sodium

Exchanges: ½ starch, 1 meat, 3 vegetable

Tomato and Goat Cheese Manicotti

8	ounces lasagna noodles (8 noodles)
2	cups 1 percent cottage cheese
2	cloves garlic, minced
$\frac{1}{4}$	cup julienned basil leaves
$\frac{1}{4}$	teaspoon kosher salt
$\frac{1}{4}$	teaspoon freshly ground black pepper
2	cups Slow-Roasted Tomatoes, chopped (see page 301)
$\frac{2}{3}$	cup low-sodium chicken broth
2	ounces soft goat cheese, divided

1. Preheat the oven to 375°F.

2. Bring a large pot of salted water to a boil. Add the noodles and cook, stirring, for 6 minutes. Drain in a single layer on paper towels.

3. In a small bowl, whisk together the cottage cheese, garlic, basil, salt, and pepper.

4. In a medium saucepan, combine the tomatoes, broth, and half of the goat cheese. Bring to a boil over medium heat.

5. Coat a small baking dish with cooking spray. Spread $\frac{1}{4}$ cup of the tomato sauce on the bottom. Spread $\frac{1}{4}$ cup of the cottage cheese mixture onto one noodle, leaving a 1" margin on one end. Roll up the pasta from the other end. Place the roll seam-side down in the dish. Repeat with the remaining noodles.

6. Pour the remaining sauce over the top, covering all surfaces, and dot with the remaining 1 ounce of goat cheese. Cover with foil and bake for 20 minutes.

Makes 8 servings

Per serving: 180 cal, 13 g pro, 26 g carb, 3 g fat, 2 g sat fat, 6 mg chol, 1 g fiber, 438 mg sodium

Exchanges: 1½ starch, ½ fat, ½ vegetable, 1 very lean meat

Harvest Lasagna

9	ounces stemmed spinach leaves		$^1/_4$	teaspoon freshly ground black pepper
1	container (15 ounces) reduced-fat ricotta cheese		$^1/_2$	cup chopped onion
$1^1/_4$	cups shredded reduced-fat mozzarella cheese		1	cup chopped bell pepper
			2	medium zucchini, chopped
$^1/_2$	cup grated Parmesan cheese		2	teaspoons minced garlic
1	egg white		1	jar (26 ounces) low-sodium tomato sauce
2	tablespoons fresh parsley, chopped			
$^1/_2$	teaspoon salt		8	no-boil lasagna noodles

1. Put the spinach in an 8" x 8" microwavable dish and cook on high for 4 minutes, or until wilted. Drain any liquid, remove the spinach from the dish and place in a bowl, and mix with the ricotta, half of the mozzarella, half of the Parmesan, the egg white, 4 teaspoons of the parsley, salt, and pepper. Wipe out the dish and generously coat it with cooking spray. Mix in the onion, pepper, zucchini, and garlic. Mix until coated with the spray, then cover tightly with microwave-safe plastic wrap and cook on high for 5 minutes, or until the vegetables are soft, stirring once. Uncover and scrape the vegetables onto a plate.

2. Spread a layer of tomato sauce over bottom of the same dish. Add a layer of two noodles. Spread a third of the cheese mixture over the noodles, covering the noodles completely. Spoon a third of the vegetable mixture over the cheese, then spoon on a quarter of the sauce, making sure the noodles are covered. Repeat the layers of noodles, cheese, vegetables, and sauce to make a total of four layers of noodles. Top the final layer with the remaining sauce. Cover with microwave-safe plastic wrap and cook on high for 10 minutes, or until the noodles are almost tender.

3. Scatter the remaining mozzarella and Parmesan over the top and cook uncovered on high for 5 minutes, or until the cheese is melted. Sprinkle with the remaining 2 teaspoons of parsley. Let sit for 5 minutes before cutting.

Makes 6 servings

Per serving: 358 cal, 24 g pro, 44 g carb, 9 g fat, 5 g sat fat, 69 mg chol, 4 g fiber, 389 mg sodium

Exchanges: 1 fat, 2 meat, 3 vegetable

Penne with Pesto alla Trapanese

¾	pound penne rigate pasta
½	pound Roma tomatoes (about 4), very ripe and sweet
8	large, fresh basil leaves
2	tablespoons unsalted roasted almonds
1	large clove garlic, peeled and crushed
¼	teaspoon red-pepper flakes
¼	teaspoon coarse sea salt or kosher salt
¼	cup extra virgin olive oil
¼	cup freshly grated Parmesan cheese (preferably Parmigiano-Reggiano or Grana Padano)

1. Cook the pasta according to the package instructions until al dente.

2. While the pasta cooks, rinse the tomatoes and basil and pat dry. Cut the tomatoes into large chunks.

3. Place the tomatoes into a blender or food processor, followed by the basil, almonds, garlic, red-pepper flakes, and salt. Blend for a minute or more to a fine puree, scraping down the sides of the bowl, and blend again if any large pieces are left.

4. With the machine still running, add the oil in a steady stream. (It will emulsify the puree into a thick pesto.)

5. Scrape the pesto into a large bowl. Drop the drained pasta onto the pesto. Toss quickly to coat the pasta, sprinkle on the cheese, and toss again. Serve immediately.

Makes 4 servings

Per serving: 496 cal, 15 g pro, 67 g carb, 19 g fat, 3 g sat fat, 4 mg chol, 4 g fiber, 231 mg sodium

Exchanges: 4½ starch, 3 fat, ½ meat, ½ vegetable

Asian Noodle Salad with Peanut Dressing

1	tablespoon low-sodium soy sauce
3	tablespoons peanut butter
2	tablespoons hoisin sauce
4	tablespoons hot water
2	tablespoons lime juice
1	teaspoon hot sauce
1	package (8.8 ounces) soba noodles
1	cup 2"-long thinly sliced zucchini spears
1	cup matchstick-cut carrots
1	cup thinly sliced red bell pepper
1	cup snow peas, ends trimmed
$\frac{1}{2}$	cup chopped green onions, green parts only
$\frac{1}{2}$	cup bean sprouts
$\frac{1}{2}$	cup chopped cilantro

1. In a blender or food processor, puree the soy sauce, peanut butter, hoisin sauce, hot water, lime juice, and hot sauce until smooth. (If the mixture is too thick, thin it with additional hot water, adding 1 tablespoon at a time.)

2. In a medium pot, cook the noodles in boiling water until tender, about 5 minutes. About 30 seconds before removing the noodles, add the zucchini and carrots. Drain, rinse briefly with cold water, and then drain again.

3. Place the cool, drained noodles, zucchini, and carrots into a large bowl. Add the pepper, snow peas, and green onions. Pour the dressing over the mixture and toss until well coated.

4. Divide the salad among four plates and garnish with the sprouts and cilantro.

Makes 4 servings

Per serving: 338 cal, 15 g pro, 61 g carb, 7 g fat, 1 g sat fat, 0 mg chol, 4 g fiber, 847 mg sodium

Exchanges: 3 starch, 1 fat, $\frac{1}{2}$ meat, 1 vegetable, $\frac{1}{2}$ very lean meat

Risotto with Squash and Pistachios

1½	tablespoons olive oil
1	cup finely chopped red onion (1 large)
1	tablespoon sugar
1	teaspoon kosher salt, divided
½	teaspoon freshly ground black pepper, divided
2	tablespoons water
1	tablespoon balsamic vinegar
1	cup Arborio rice
4½	cups low-sodium chicken broth, divided
4	cups Roasted Butternut Squash (See recipe on page 302.)
1	ounce soft goat cheese
¼	cup unsalted, dry-roasted, shelled, chopped pistachios
¼	cup fresh mint, thinly sliced

1. In a large pan, heat the oil over medium heat and sauté the onion for 10 minutes, until soft. Sprinkle with the sugar, ½ teaspoon of the salt, and ¼ teaspoon of the pepper. Sauté 3 minutes longer, until browned. Add the water and vinegar to the pan and sauté until all the liquid has evaporated, about 2 to 3 minutes.

2. Stir in the rice and cook for 2 minutes. Add 1 cup of the broth and stir constantly until the broth is absorbed, for 3 to 5 minutes. Stir in the squash and 2½ cups of the broth and bring to a vigorous simmer, about 5 to 7 minutes. Reduce the heat to medium-low and cook for 15 minutes, stirring every 5 minutes. Stir in the remaining 1 cup of broth and cook until the rice is soft, about 6 to 8 minutes. Stir in the cheese until melted, 1 minute longer.

3. Remove from the heat, mound onto serving plates, and sprinkle the pistachios and mint over the top.

Makes 8 servings

Per serving: 241 cal, 7 g pro, 39 g carb, 8 g fat, 2 g sat fat, 4 mg chol, 4 g fiber, 459 mg sodium

Exchanges: 1 starch, 1 fat, ½ meat, 2½ vegetable

Red Pepper Pesto Pizza

See photo insert.

3	tablespoons reduced-fat ricotta cheese
1	teaspoon ready-made roasted garlic
1	ready-made flatbread, such as Flatout, or whole wheat pita
1	tablespoon ready-made pesto
2	tablespoons ready-made roasted red peppers
3	tablespoons grated reduced-fat mozzarella cheese
	Dash of freshly ground black pepper

1. Preheat the oven to 375°F.

2. In a small bowl, stir together the ricotta cheese and garlic, blending well. Spread the mixture on the flatbread or pita. Top with dollops of the pesto, bell peppers, and mozzarella. Season with the pepper.

3. Place on a baking sheet and bake for 6 minutes.

Makes 1 serving

Per serving: 298 cal, 22 g pro, 23 g carb, 15 g fat, 5 g sat fat, 28 mg chol, 9 g fiber, 768 mg sodium

Exchanges: 1½ fat, 1½ meat, ½ vegetable

CHICKEN AND TURKEY MAIN DISHES

Lemon Herb Chicken

2	tablespoons + 4 teaspoons olive oil
2	large chicken breasts
	Juice and zest of 1 lemon
$\frac{1}{3}$	cup fresh parsley
$\frac{1}{3}$	cup fresh mint
$\frac{1}{3}$	cup fresh basil
	Salt
	Freshly ground black pepper
$\frac{1}{3}$	cup white wine

1. Preheat the oven to 400°F.

2. In an ovenproof skillet, heat 2 tablespoons of the oil over high heat. Place the chicken in the skillet and sear for 2 minutes per side.

3. Meanwhile, place the remaining 4 teaspoons of oil, along with the lemon juice, zest, parsley, mint, and basil, into a blender or food processor and pulse until well mixed.

4. Roast the chicken for 8 minutes. Remove the skillet from the oven and place the chicken onto a plate. Season with salt and pepper to taste, and then pour the wine into the skillet, scraping up any brown bits from the bottom of the pan. Add the herb sauce to the skillet and cook on the stovetop for 1 minute, stirring frequently. Pour the sauce over the chicken.

Makes 2 servings

Per serving: 377 cal, 28 g pro, 5 g carb, 24 g fat, 4 g sat fat, 68 mg chol, 1 g fiber, 164 mg sodium

Exchanges: 4½ fat, 4 very lean meat

5-Minute Chicken Salad Sandwich

1	rib celery, finely chopped
1	tablespoon finely chopped onion
1	tablespoon pine nuts
1	heaping teaspoon spicy brown mustard
1	heaping teaspoon fat-free sour cream
1	heaping teaspoon plain yogurt
	Pinch of freshly ground black pepper
2	cans (3 ounces each) chunk chicken, rinsed and drained twice
4	slices whole-grain bread
2	leaves lettuce

1. In a large bowl, mix together the celery, onion, pine nuts, mustard, sour cream, yogurt, and pepper. Add the chicken and toss lightly.

2. Divide the salad, spreading each half onto a slice of bread. Top each with a lettuce leaf and another bread slice.

Makes 2 servings

Per serving: 267 cal, 28 g pro, 31 g carb, 6 g fat, 0 g sat fat, 38 mg chol, 11 g fiber, 495 mg sodium

Exchanges: 1½ starch, ½ fat, ½ vegetable, 1 meat

Coconut Curried Chicken

1	cup jasmine or basmati rice
1½	cups low-sodium chicken broth
1	pound boneless, skinless chicken thighs, cut into bite-size pieces
1	small onion, thickly sliced, then halved
1	medium red bell pepper, cut into strips
2	teaspoons minced garlic
2	teaspoons minced fresh ginger
½	teaspoon salt
⅔	cup canned light coconut milk
1	tablespoon red curry paste
1	tablespoon chopped fresh basil, preferably Thai

1. In a 2-quart microwavable bowl, combine the rice and broth. Cover tightly with microwave-safe plastic wrap and cook on high for 5 minutes. Reduce to 50 percent power and cook for 18 to 20 minutes, or until tender. Set aside.

2. Generously coat a 2-quart microwavable dish with cooking spray. Mix in the chicken, onion, pepper, garlic, ginger, and salt. Cover tightly and microwave on high for 3 to 5 minutes, or until the vegetables are soft.

3. In a cup, mix the coconut milk and curry paste. Pour over the chicken and cook, uncovered, on high for 8 minutes, or until the chicken is no longer pink.

4. Serve with the rice garnished with the basil.

Makes 4 servings

Per serving: 286 cal, 27 g pro, 25 g carb, 8 g fat, 3 g sat fat, 96 mg chol, 1 g fiber, 595 mg sodium

Exchanges: 1 starch, ½ fat, ½ vegetable, 3 very lean meat

Grilled Chicken with Goat Cheese and Apples

See photo insert.

1	large Braeburn apple, julienned
¼	cup sliced sweet onion
1	tablespoon apple cider vinegar
1	tablespoon extra virgin olive oil
1	tablespoon finely chopped mint leaves
½	teaspoon julienned jalapeño chile (Wear plastic gloves when handling.)
2	ounces soft goat cheese, crumbled
½	teaspoon kosher salt
⅛	teaspoon freshly ground black pepper
⅛	teaspoon ground red pepper
⅛	teaspoon ground cumin
4	boneless, skinless chicken breast halves (6 ounces each)

1. Preheat the grill to medium-high.

2. In a small bowl, mix together the apple, onion, vinegar, oil, mint, and chile. Stir in the cheese, cover, and chill.

3. In another small bowl, combine the salt, black pepper, red pepper, and cumin. Sprinkle onto the chicken. Grill for 12 to 16 minutes, flipping once, until cooked through.

4. Top each breast with 2 tablespoons of the apple-cheese mixture.

Makes 4 servings

Per serving: 276 cal, 37 g pro, 7 g carb, 11 g fat, 4 g sat fat, 101 mg chol, 1 g fiber, 378 mg sodium

Exchanges: 1½ fat, ½ meat, ½ vegetable, 5 very lean meat

Chicken Spinach Parm

See photo insert.

1	tablespoon olive oil
2	boneless, skinless chicken breasts
2	tablespoons Italian-seasoned bread crumbs
2	teaspoons grated Parmesan cheese
	Salt
	Freshly ground black pepper
2	small cloves garlic, crushed
½	cup low-sodium marinara
6	handfuls baby spinach leaves (about 6 cups)

1. In a nonstick skillet, heat the oil over medium heat.

2. Meanwhile, pound the chicken to ¼" thickness, then sprinkle with the bread crumbs and cheese and season with salt and pepper to taste, pressing so the crumbs stick. Place in the skillet, add the garlic and sauté for 2 to 3 minutes per side. Add the marinara, and heat for 2 minutes. Add the spinach, turning frequently with tongs until it wilts, about 6 minutes.

Makes 2 servings

Per serving: 280 cal, 31 g pro, 17 g carb, 10 g fat, 2 g sat fat, 70 mg chol, 4 g fiber, 478 mg sodium

Exchanges: ½ starch, 1½ fat, 2 vegetable, 4 very lean meat

Spicy Chicken Stir-Fry

1	tablespoon peanut oil
1/2	teaspoon red-pepper flakes
2	thin-cut, boneless, skinless chicken breasts, cut into bite-size pieces or strips
2/3	cup asparagus tips
2/3	cup thinly sliced carrots
1/2	medium onion, cut into bite-size pieces or strips
2/3	cup frozen snow peas
2	tablespoons sliced almonds
2	teaspoons reduced-sodium soy sauce

1. In a medium skillet, combine the peanut oil and red-pepper flakes. Heat over medium-high heat.

2. Add the chicken and cook for 2 to 3 minutes, stirring frequently. Add the remaining ingredients and cook for another 2 to 3 minutes, still stirring often.

Makes 2 servings

Per serving: 277 cal, 31 g pro, 12 g carb, 12 g fat, 2 g sat fat, 68 mg chol, 4 g fiber, 286 mg sodium

Exchanges: 2 fat, 2 vegetable, 4 very lean meat

Pan-Fried Chicken with Tarragon

2	tablespoons lemon juice
2	tablespoons olive oil
$\frac{1}{2}$	teaspoon Dijon mustard
$\frac{1}{8}$	teaspoon salt plus more to taste (optional)
1	pound chicken breast tenders (12 to 16 tenders)
2	tablespoons poultry seasoning
1	tablespoon dried tarragon, crumbled
1	tablespoon dried garlic
8	cups (5 ounces) loosely packed baby salad greens

1. In a large bowl, whisk together the lemon juice, oil, and mustard and salt to taste. Set aside.

2. Place the chicken between two sheets of plastic wrap. With a kitchen mallet (or the bottom of a small, heavy saucepan), pound the tenders 2 or 3 times until they are $\frac{1}{4}$" thick.

3. In a medium bowl, mix the poultry seasoning, tarragon, garlic, and 1 to 2 pinches of salt. Coat the chicken with the mixture.

4. Coat a large nonstick skillet with cooking spray and place on high heat. When the skillet is hot, add 4 to 5 chicken tenders and cook on medium-high until golden and firm, 1 to 2 minutes per side. Wipe down the pan with a paper towel to remove any burned crumbs and repeat the process until all the tenders are cooked.

5. Add the greens to the large bowl and toss with the dressing.

6. To serve, place 2 cups of the greens on dinner plates and top with 3 or 4 chicken tenders.

Makes 4 servings

Per serving: 190 cal, 27 g pro, 6 g carb, 8 g fat, 1 g sat fat, 67 mg chol, 2 g fiber, 147 mg sodium

Exchanges: 1½ fat, ½ vegetable, 3 very lean meat

Chicken Spinach Pizza

2	ready-made flatbread (We used Flatout.)
6	tablespoons low-sodium marinara sauce
$^2/_3$	cup frozen spinach, defrosted and thoroughly drained
$^1/_2$	cup crumbled feta cheese
$1^1/_2$	cups chopped precooked chicken
2	tablespoons sliced fresh basil
	Dash of salt
	Dash of freshly ground black pepper

1. Preheat the oven to 375°F.

2. Place the flatbread onto a baking sheet. Spread the marinara over the flatbread. Top with the spinach, cheese, chicken, and basil. Season to taste with salt and pepper. Bake for 6 minutes.

Makes 2 servings

Per serving: 340 cal, 41 g pro, 12 g carb, 12 g fat, 7 g sat fat, 123 mg chol, 3 g fiber, 753 mg sodium

Exchanges: ½ starch, 1½ fat, 1 meat, 1 vegetable, 4½ very lean meat

Tuscan Chicken Pasta

2	ounces penne pasta (We used Barilla Plus.)
2	chicken breasts, pounded to $1/4$" thickness
	Salt
	Freshly ground black pepper
1	teaspoon olive oil
1	clove garlic, crushed
$1/2$	teaspoon dried rosemary
1	cup cannellini beans, rinsed
2	tablespoons diced roasted red pepper
4	cups baby spinach leaves
2	tablespoons grated Parmesan cheese

1. Cook the pasta according to the package directions.

2. While the pasta is boiling, season the chicken on each side with salt and black pepper to taste. Sear it in a skillet over medium-high heat for 3 to 4 minutes a side. Remove the chicken from the skillet and set aside.

3. Add the oil, garlic, rosemary, beans, red pepper, and spinach to the skillet. Cook, turning frequently, until the spinach wilts, for 1 to 2 minutes.

4. Slice the chicken, drain the pasta, and toss with the bean mixture. Spoon the pasta into two bowls and top each with 1 tablespoon of Parmesan.

Makes 2 servings

Per serving: 405 cal, 40 g pro, 46 g carb, 6 g fat, 2 g sat fat, 73 mg chol, 9 g fiber, 633 mg sodium

Exchanges: 2½ starch, ½ fat, ½ meat, 1 vegetable, 4 very lean meat

Turkey Meat Loaf

$\frac{1}{2}$	pound ground sirloin
$\frac{1}{2}$	pound ground turkey breast
2	eggs
1	cup whole wheat crackers, crushed
$\frac{3}{4}$	cup diced onion
2	cloves garlic, crushed
$\frac{1}{2}$	teaspoon dried oregano
$\frac{1}{2}$	cup barbecue sauce, plus extra

1. Preheat the oven to 350°F.

2. In a large bowl, mix the beef and turkey until well blended. Add the eggs. Mix in the remaining ingredients, including the half cup of barbecue sauce, until well blended.

3. Form the meat mixture into a loaf shape and place it onto a broiler pan. Coat it with the extra barbecue sauce.

4. Bake for 1 hour. Double-check the internal temperature with a meat thermometer; it should read 160°F.

Makes 4 servings

Per serving: 424 cal, 41 g pro, 40 g carb, 11 g fat, 3 g sat fat, 146 mg chol, 4 g fiber, 765 mg sodium

Exchanges: 1½ starch, ½ other carbohydrate, 1 fat, ½ meat, ½ vegetable, 5 very lean meat

Turkey Burgers

See photo insert.

10	ounces ground turkey, divided into two patties
	Salt
	Freshly ground black pepper
2	tablespoons low-sodium teriyaki sauce
2	slices fresh pineapple
2	thick slices red onion
2	whole wheat buns, toasted
$\frac{1}{2}$	jalapeño chile, thinly sliced (Wear plastic gloves when handling.)
2	slices Swiss cheese

1. Take the meat out of the refrigerator 1 hour before cooking. Season it with salt and pepper. Preheat the grill.

2. Grill the burgers over high heat for 3 to 4 minutes a side, basting occasionally with the teriyaki sauce.

3. While the burgers cook, grill the pineapple and onion until lightly charred. Put each burger onto a bun and layer on onion, pineapple, chile, and cheese.

Makes 2 servings

Per serving: 348 cal, 4 g pro, 42 g carb, 4 g fat, 0.4 g sat fat, 56 mg chol, 6 g fiber, 552 mg sodium

Exchanges: 1½ starch, ½ fruit, 2 vegetable, 4 very lean meat

Jambalaya

2	links turkey sausage, sliced, or 2 ounces loose sausage
3	ribs celery, chopped
1	medium onion, chopped
1	green bell pepper, chopped
3	cloves garlic, minced
1	teaspoon ground red pepper
1	teaspoon dried thyme
	Salt
	Freshly ground black pepper
2	cans (14.5 ounces each) no-salt-added diced tomatoes with juice
2	cups reduced-sodium chicken broth
1	cup long-grain brown rice
1	pound boneless, skinless chicken breast, cut into 1" pieces
	Dash hot sauce (optional)

1. Heat a large saucepan coated with cooking spray on medium-high heat. Add the turkey sausage. Cook until golden.

2. Add the celery, onion, bell pepper, and garlic. Sauté until tender, 5 to 7 minutes. Reduce the heat, and add the red pepper and thyme as well as the salt and black pepper to taste. Cook for 3 to 5 more minutes.

3. Add the tomatoes with juice, broth, and rice. Bring to a boil. Turn down the heat and cover.

4. Let simmer for about 45 minutes, until the liquid is absorbed and the rice is tender. Add the chicken in the last 30 minutes of cooking time. Add hot sauce, if desired.

Makes 4 servings

Per serving: 410 cal, 38 g pro, 51 g carb, 5 g fat, 1 g sat fat, 77 mg chol, 5 g fiber, 418 mg sodium

Exchanges: 2½ starch, ½ meat, 3½ vegetable, 4 very lean meat

BEEF, PORK, LAMB, AND MORE MAIN DISHES

Apple, Gouda, and Crispy Prosciutto Panini

See photo insert.

2	ounces prosciutto
4	teaspoons honey Dijon mustard
8	$\frac{1}{2}$" slices whole-grain baguette (about 6 ounces total)
2	medium McIntosh apples, halved, cored, and thinly sliced lengthwise
2	ounces light Gouda cheese, thinly sliced

1. Heat a large nonstick skillet over medium heat and cook the prosciutto for 8 minutes, turning occasionally, until crispy. Remove from the pan and set aside on a paper towel.

2. Spread the mustard on 4 slices of the bread. Lay one-quarter of the apples (about 10 slices) atop the mustard on each bread slice. Top each with one-quarter of the prosciutto and cheese and 1 slice of the remaining bread. Lightly coat both sides of the sandwiches with cooking spray.

3. Heat the same skillet over medium heat and toast the sandwiches for 4 to 5 minutes per side, pressing down with a spatula often, until golden brown on both sides and the cheese is melted.

Makes 4 servings

Per serving: 224 cal, 13 g pro, 33 g carb, 5 g fat, 2 g sat fat, 17 mg chol, 3 g fiber, 826 mg sodium

Exchanges: 1½ starch, ½ fruit, ½ meat

Panzanella with Tomatoes, White Beans, Basil, and Prosciutto

See photo insert.

4	thick slices crusty whole-grain bread, cut into 1½" pieces (about 4 cups)
1	can (15 ounces) cannellini beans, rinsed and drained
1	cup basil leaves, torn
1	pound cherry tomatoes, halved
2	tablespoons extra virgin olive oil
2	tablespoons balsamic vinegar
	Salt
4	thin slices prosciutto

1. Preheat the oven to 450°F. Coat a baking sheet with cooking spray.

2. Place the bread cubes onto the baking sheet and spritz bread with cooking spray. Bake until lightly toasted, 3 to 4 minutes, shaking once or twice to heat evenly.

3. Meanwhile, in a large bowl, toss the beans, basil, tomatoes, oil, and vinegar and salt to taste until combined. Set aside.

4. Cut the prosciutto into tiny pieces using kitchen shears. Cook in a nonstick skillet on medium-high heat until crispy. Remove and drain on paper towels.

5. Add the toasted bread to the tomato mixture and toss lightly. Divide among four plates and garnish with the prosciutto.

Makes 4 servings

Per serving: 293 cal, 11 g pro, 42 g carb, 9 g fat, 1 g sat fat, 3 mg chol, 7 g fiber, 510 mg sodium

Exchanges: 2½ starch, 1½ fat, 1 vegetable

Grilled Italian Skirt Steak

1	large red onion, sliced
1	tablespoon olive oil, divided
2	tablespoons balsamic vinegar
2	cloves garlic, minced
1	can (15.5 ounces) cannellini beans
1	tablespoon fresh chopped rosemary or 1 teaspoon dried rosemary
	Salt (optional)
	Freshly ground black pepper (optional)
	Juice of $\frac{1}{2}$ lemon
12	ounces skirt or flank steak

1. In a medium pan over medium heat, cook the onion in half of the oil for 10 minutes, until it's soft and slightly brown. Add the vinegar and cook another 5 minutes.

2. Heat a pot with the remaining oil over medium heat. Add the garlic, beans, and rosemary and cook for 5 minutes. Use a potato masher or a fork to roughly mash the beans. Add the salt, pepper, and lemon juice to taste.

3. Heat a grill, grill pan, or cast-iron skillet over high heat. Season the steak with salt and pepper and grill for 3 to 4 minutes per side for medium rare. Slice and serve over the beans, and spoon the onions on top.

Makes 2 servings

Per serving: 744 cal, 62 g pro, 60 g carb, 28 g fat, 9 g sat fat, 102 mg chol, 12 g fiber, 147 mg sodium

Exchanges: 3 starch, 2 fat, 6 meat, 1 vegetable

Nuke-and-Eat Asian Stir-Fry

1	egg, beaten		2	carrots, sliced into 2" strips
4	tablespoons low-sodium soy sauce		1	can (8 ounces) sliced water
1	pound beef sirloin, sliced into			chestnuts, drained
	2" strips		1	medium onion, sliced
1	tablespoon cornstarch		1	bunch green onions, sliced into
$\frac{1}{2}$	teaspoon red pepper flakes			2" strips
1	tablespoon sesame oil		10	ounces cooked Rice Expressions
1	tablespoon chopped garlic			Organic Brown Rice (See note.)
2	teaspoons grated fresh ginger			

1. In a bowl, combine the egg and 1 tablespoon of the soy sauce, and stir well. Then add the sirloin strips and set aside to marinate.

2. In another bowl, mix the remaining soy sauce, the cornstarch, and the red pepper flakes. Set aside.

3. In a large nonstick skillet, heat the oil over medium-high heat. Stir-fry the garlic and ginger for about 30 seconds, stirring constantly. Then, at 30-second intervals, individually add the carrots, water chestnuts, onion, and green onions.

4. Remove all the vegetables from the skillet and place them into a bowl. Put the beef-marinade mixture in the skillet, cook for 2 to 3 minutes, then pour in the sauce, stirring and cooking until it's thick and bubbly.

5. Add the vegetables back to the skillet, and cook everything together for a couple of minutes, or until hot. Serve over the rice.

Makes 3 servings

Note: This frozen rice is precooked and packaged in individual microwavable pouches. You can buy it at riceexpressions.com.

Per serving: 477 cal, 41 g pro, 46 g carb, 14 g fat, 4 g sat fat, 142 mg chol, 7 g fiber, 866 mg sodium

Exchanges: $1\frac{1}{2}$ starch, 1 fat, 4 meat, 3 vegetable

Beef and Broccoli over Brown Rice

1½	cups brown rice	4	green onions, cut into 1" pieces
8	ounces beef fillet	1	ounce ginger, cut into long strips
	Salt	2	cups cut-up broccoli or broccolini
	Freshly ground black pepper		(1" pieces)
3	tablespoons canola oil	½	cup chicken or beef broth (can
3	tablespoons diced shallots		substitute white wine or water)
3	tablespoons diced garlic	2	tablespoons balsamic vinegar
1	tablespoon fermented black beans		
	(or black bean paste)		

1. Cook the rice per the package directions.

2. Meanwhile, heat a cast-iron pan or wok over high heat. Season the beef with salt and pepper to taste. Sear on one side for 3 minutes, then flip and sear for another 3 minutes. Remove to a cutting board and let rest for about 5 minutes.

3. Heat a wok or deep sauté pan over high heat. Add the oil, then the shallots, garlic, and fermented black beans. Reduce the heat to medium and cook, stirring occasionally, for 2 to 3 minutes until fragrant.

4. Add the green onions and ginger. Stir-fry for an additional 2 minutes. Add the broccoli or broccolini, broth, and vinegar. Cover, turn the heat to high, and cook for 2 minutes. Season with salt and pepper to taste. Transfer to a serving dish.

5. Cut the beef into thin slices and arrange on top of the broccoli mixture. Serve immediately over the rice.

Makes 4 servings

Per serving: 484 cal, 21 g pro, 63 g carbs, 17 g fat, 3 g sat fat, 38 mg chol, 4 g fiber, 131 mg sodium

Exchanges: 3½ starch, 3 fat, 1 vegetable, 2 very lean meat

Mini Pita Burgers with Cucumber Mint Salad

See photo insert.

1	tablespoon mayonnaise		$1^1/_2$	teaspoons cumin
1	tablespoon lemon juice		1	teaspoon dried garlic
$^1/_4$	cup chopped mint		1	teaspoon paprika
	Kosher salt (optional)		1	teaspoon coriander
2	large cucumbers, peeled and thinly sliced		1–2	pinches salt
			1	pound lean ground beef
$^1/_4$	cup grated onion (1 small)		4	whole wheat pitas (6" diameters), halved
$^1/_4$	cup chopped parsley			

1. Preheat the grill.

2. In a medium bowl, whisk together the mayonnaise, lemon juice, and mint and kosher salt (if using) to taste. Add the cucumbers and toss. Set aside.

3. Place the onion, parsley, cumin, garlic, paprika, coriander, and salt in a medium bowl and stir until thoroughly combined.

4. Add the beef and blend the mixture into the meat with your hands. (Don't overhandle the meat or the burgers will get tough.)

5. Form the beef into 16 mini patties and grill until cooked through, 3 to 4 minutes per side.

6. Meanwhile, lightly warm the pitas in a toaster.

7. To serve, stuff each pita pocket with 4 or 5 cucumber slices and 2 burgers and drizzle with the juices from the salad. Serve the remaining salad on the side.

Makes 4 servings

Per serving: 330 cal, 30 g pro, 34 g carb, 9 g fat, 2 g sat fat, 61 mg chol, 6 g fiber, 441 mg sodium

Exchanges: 1 fat, 1 vegetable, 3 very lean meat

Stuffed Peppers

4	bell peppers (green, yellow, or red)
1/4	teaspoon extra virgin olive oil
1	pound extra-lean ground beef
1	egg white
1/2	cup finely chopped yellow onion
2	tablespoons canned corn
1	tablespoon finely chopped fresh parsley
	Pinch of freshly ground black pepper
3/4	cup low-sodium tomato or spaghetti sauce, divided
1	teaspoon prepared horseradish

1. Preheat the oven to 375°F.

2. Cut the tops off the bell peppers, carefully remove the seeds and white membranes, and discard them. Lightly coat the outside of the peppers with the oil.

3. In a large bowl, combine the beef, egg white, onion, corn, parsley, black pepper, and 1/4 cup of the sauce. Stuff the mixture into the 4 peppers, dividing it evenly.

4. Pour 1/4" of water into a 9" × 13" baking pan and add the peppers, cut side up. Bake for 40 minutes.

5. Remove the peppers. Combine the horseradish and the remaining 1/2 cup of tomato sauce and add a little of the mixture to the top of each pepper. Bake for another 10 minutes.

Makes 4 servings

Per serving: 195 cal, 25 g pro, 14 g carb, 5 g fat, 2 g sat fat, 60 mg chol, 4 g fiber, 111 mg sodium

Exchanges: 1/2 fat, 1 1/2 vegetable, 3 1/2 very lean meat

Jerk Pork with Pineapple and Black Beans

See photo insert.

$1\frac{1}{2}$	pounds sweet potatoes (about 2)
4	bone-in pork loin chops (about 1" thick), trimmed of fat
$2\frac{1}{2}$	tablespoons Jamaican jerk seasoning, divided
1	can (8 ounces) pineapple bits
$\frac{1}{2}$	cup chopped red bell pepper
2	green onions, chopped
2	tablespoons brown sugar
2	tablespoons cider vinegar
1	can (15 ounces) black beans, rinsed and drained
1	tablespoon extra virgin olive oil

1. Prick the potato skins with a fork and microwave on high for 13 to 15 minutes, or until soft. Set aside.

2. Season the chops with 2 tablespoons of the jerk seasoning and arrange in a 3-quart microwavable dish with the bones facing outward.

3. In a large bowl, mix the pineapple (with half of the juice), pepper, green onions, sugar, and vinegar. Pour evenly over the chops. Cover tightly with microwave-safe plastic wrap and cook on high for 6 minutes.

4. Rotate the chops and scatter the beans in the dish. Re-cover and cook on high for 5 to 6 minutes, or until the chops are barely pink in the center and register 145°F on an instant-read thermometer.

5. Cut each potato in half and drizzle with the oil and remaining jerk seasoning. Serve alongside the chops.

Makes 4 servings

Per serving: 457 cal, 26 g pro, 67 g carb, 9 g fat, 2 g sat fat, 47 mg chol, 11 g fiber, 907 mg sodium

Exchanges: 3 starch, ½ fruit, ½ other carbohydrate, 1½ fat, ½ vegetable, 2½ very lean meat

Pork Souvlaki

1	tablespoon extra virgin olive oil
1	tablespoon lemon juice
1	teaspoon dried oregano, divided
1	teaspoon kosher salt, divided
2	pinches freshly ground black pepper, divided
2	pounds boneless pork loin roast, trimmed and cut into 1" cubes

1. Preheat the grill or broiler to high.

2. In a small bowl, whisk together the oil, lemon juice, $\frac{1}{2}$ teaspoon of the oregano, $\frac{1}{2}$ teaspoon of the salt, and 1 pinch of the pepper and set aside.

3. Thread the pork cubes onto 12 skewers (if using wooden skewers, soak them in water for 30 minutes beforehand). Sprinkle the skewers with the remaining $\frac{1}{2}$ teaspoon of oregano, $\frac{1}{2}$ teaspoon of salt, and 1 pinch of the pepper.

4. Grill the souvlaki for 8 to 10 minutes, turning occasionally, until browned and just cooked through. Remove from the heat and brush generously with the oil mixture on all sides.

Makes 6 servings

Per serving: 236 cal, 33 g pro, 0 g carb, 10 g fat, 3 g sat fat, 83 mg chol, 0 g fiber, 388 mg sodium

Exchanges: 1½ fat, 4½ very lean meat

Apple-Topped Chops

1	tablespoon olive oil
2	small cloves garlic, crushed
2	thin-cut boneless pork chops (3 ounces each)
2	small red apples, such as Gala or Red Delicious, cored and diced
4	teaspoons balsamic or red wine vinegar
2	tablespoons bourbon
2	tablespoons grainy mustard
	Salt
	Freshly ground black pepper

1. Combine the oil and garlic in a nonstick skillet over medium-high heat. Place the pork chops in the center of the skillet.

2. In a medium bowl, toss the apple with the vinegar and bourbon, and then add the mixture to the skillet between the pork and the edges of the pan. Cook for 6 minutes, turning the pork once and the apple pieces a few times. When ready to serve, top the pork with mustard. Season to taste with salt and pepper.

Makes 2 servings

Per serving: 338 cal, 20 g pro, 18 g carb, 18 g fat, 5 g sat fat, 59 mg chol, 3 g fiber, 328 mg sodium

Exchanges: 1 fruit, ½ other carbohydrate, 2 fat, 2½ meat

Pita Pizza

4	tablespoons marinara sauce
2	whole wheat pitas (6" diameter)
2	tablespoons Italian seasoning (or dried basil and oregano)
$\frac{1}{2}$	cup diced pineapple
2	slices lean, low-sodium ham
$\frac{1}{2}$	cup shredded low-fat mozzarella cheese

1. Preheat the oven to 425°F.

2. Spread the marinara sauce over the pitas, add the Italian seasoning, and top with the pineapple, ham, and cheese. Place them on a baking sheet and bake for 8 minutes on the center oven rack.

Makes 2 servings

Per serving: 287 cal, 17 g pro, 44 g carb, 7 g fat, 3 g sat fat, 18 mg chol, 6 g fiber, 790 mg sodium

Exchanges: 2 starch, $\frac{1}{2}$ fruit, $\frac{1}{2}$ fat, $1\frac{1}{2}$ meat

Turkish Lamb with Pistachio Couscous

1	box (6 ounces) garlic-herb couscous
1¼	cups warm water
⅓	cup pistachio nuts, shells removed
1½	tablespoons lemon-pepper seasoning salt
1	tablespoon dried thyme
1	teaspoon sugar
1	teaspoon ground cardamom
1	teaspoon ground turmeric
½	teaspoon saffron threads, crushed
1¼	pounds boneless leg of lamb, cut into 1" cubes
1	cup chopped onion
2	teaspoons minced garlic
1	tablespoon fresh minced ginger
½	cup raisins
2	cups fresh or canned tomatoes, chopped

1. Combine the couscous spice bag and water in a 2-quart microwavable bowl. Cover tightly and cook on high for 6 to 7 minutes, or until simmering. Remove and stir in the couscous and pistachios. Cover and let stand for 8 minutes.

2. Meanwhile, in a 2-quart microwavable dish, mix the lemon-pepper, thyme, sugar, cardamom, turmeric, and saffron. Add the lamb and toss to coat.

3. Mix in the onion, garlic, and ginger. Cook on high for 5 to 6 minutes, or until the vegetables are soft, stirring once halfway through.

4. Stir in the raisins and tomatoes, cover tightly with microwave-safe plastic wrap, and cook on high for 5 to 7 minutes, or until the lamb is no longer pink. Serve with the couscous.

Makes 4 servings

Per serving: 516 cal, 39 g pro, 60 g carb, 15 g fat, 4 g sat fat, 91 mg chol, 6 g fiber, 984 mg sodium

Exchanges: 2 starch, 1 fruit, 2 fat, 1½ vegetable, 4½ very lean meat

FISH AND SEAFOOD MAIN DISHES

Mediterranean Roasted Cod

1	pint cherry tomatoes
½	bulb fennel or yellow onion, sliced thin
½	tablespoon extra virgin olive oil
	Salt
	Freshly ground black pepper
2	tablespoons prepared olive tapenade, divided
2	6-ounce cod, halibut, or snapper fillets
1	cup couscous
4	tablespoons pine nuts
4	tablespoons chopped fresh basil

1. Preheat the oven to 400°F.

2. Lay the tomatoes and fennel on a baking dish and toss with the oil and salt and pepper to taste. Slather 1 tablespoon of the tapenade onto each fish fillet and lay the fillets in the baking dish with the vegetables. Roast for 10 to 12 minutes, until the tomatoes are soft and the flesh of the fish flakes with gentle pressure from your finger.

3. In a medium bowl, combine the couscous, pine nuts, and basil. Serve with the fish.

Makes 2 servings

Per serving: 469 cal, 46 g pro, 32 g carb, 18 g fat, 2 g sat fat, 94 mg chol, 6 g fiber, 830 mg sodium

Exchanges: 1 starch, 3 fat, 2 vegetable, 5½ very lean meat

Grilled Halibut with Roasted-Tomato Tapenade

See photo insert.

$\frac{1}{2}$	cup Slow-Roasted Tomatoes, chopped (See recipe on page 301.)
3	kalamata olives, pitted and finely chopped
1	tablespoon drained capers, finely chopped
1	tablespoon finely chopped red onion
1	teaspoon red wine vinegar
1	pound halibut
$1\frac{1}{2}$	teaspoons olive oil
$\frac{1}{4}$	teaspoon kosher salt
$\frac{1}{4}$	teaspoon freshly ground black pepper

1. In a small bowl, combine the tomatoes, olives, capers, onion, and vinegar. Set aside.

2. Preheat the grill to medium. Brush the halibut with the oil to lightly coat, and season with the salt and pepper. Grill 6 to 10 minutes, turning once, or until the center of the fish is just opaque.

3. Spoon the tapenade over the top of the fish.

Makes 4 servings

Per serving: 167 cal, 24 g pro, 2 g carb, 6 g fat, 1 g sat fat, 36 mg chol, 1 g fiber, 353 mg sodium

Exchanges: $\frac{1}{2}$ fat, $\frac{1}{2}$ vegetable, $3\frac{1}{2}$ very lean meat

Whole Roasted Fish with Lemon and Oregano

1	tablespoon extra virgin olive oil
2	teaspoons freshly squeezed lemon juice
½	teaspoon dried oregano
¼	teaspoon freshly ground black pepper
1	teaspoon kosher salt, divided
2	whole sea bass (1¼ pounds each), cleaned by fishmonger
2	cloves garlic, sliced
8	thin slices lemon

1. Preheat the grill or broiler to medium-high and coat the rack lightly with cooking spray.

2. In a small bowl, whisk together the oil, lemon juice, oregano, pepper, and ½ teaspoon of the salt. Set aside.

3. Make three shallow vertical slits along each side of the fish and rub with the remaining ½ teaspoon of salt. Brush the inside of the fish with the oil mixture and stuff with the garlic and lemon.

4. Grill the fish for 16 to 20 minutes, turning and basting twice with the remaining oil mixture, until the fish is golden brown and the flesh begins to turn opaque. Let the fish rest for 10 minutes before serving.

Makes 4 servings

Per serving: 237 cal, 38 g pro, 2 g carb, 8 g fat, 2 g sat fat, 84 mg chol, 1 g fiber, 621 mg sodium

Exchanges: 1 fat, 5½ very lean meat

Spicy Sea Bass in a Flash

$^1/_2$	tablespoon olive oil
2	6-ounce fillets of sea bass, cod, or other firm white fish
	Salt
	Freshly ground black pepper
$^1/_2$	cup white wine
1	small onion, sliced
$^1/_2$	cup pitted, chopped green olives
1	can (12 ounces) whole peeled tomatoes
2	cloves garlic, minced
1	teaspoon red pepper flakes

1. Heat a large sauté pan over medium-high heat. Add the oil.

2. Season the fish with salt and black pepper. When the oil is hot, add the fillets flesh side down and cook for 3 minutes, until a crust has formed. Remove the fish from the pan and set aside.

3. Add the wine and onion to the pan and cook for 3 minutes. Add the olives, tomatoes, garlic, and red pepper flakes and cook for another 3 minutes. Season with salt and pepper to taste.

4. Return the fish to the pan. Baste the fillets with the simmering tomato sauce. Cook until the flesh flakes with gentle pressure, for 5 to 7 minutes.

Makes 2 servings

Per serving: 373 cal, 34 g pro, 16 g carb, 15 g fat, 2 g sat fat, 70 mg chol, 3 g fiber, 900 mg sodium

Exchanges: $^1/_2$ other carbohydrate, $2^1/_2$ fat, $1^1/_2$ vegetable, $4^1/_2$ very lean meat

Cedar-Plank Salmon with Spicy Cucumbers

1	large, untreated cedar plank
2	tablespoons fresh mint or cilantro, chopped
1	large English cucumber, seeded and sliced
2	tablespoons rice wine vinegar
1	teaspoon red-pepper flakes
2	teaspoons sesame seeds + more for garnish
	Salt
	Freshly ground black pepper
	Olive oil
2	6-ounce salmon fillets

1. Soak the cedar plank in water for at least 2 hours.

2. In a medium bowl, combine the mint or cilantro, cucumber, rice wine vinegar, red-pepper flakes, and 2 teaspoons of the sesame seeds. Season to taste with salt and black pepper.

3. Clean a grill or grill pan thoroughly. Next, rub the grates with an oil-soaked paper towel. Preheat over high heat. Lay the cedar plank on the grill. Season the salmon with salt and pepper. When the plank begins to smoke, lay the fillets on it, skin side down. Close the top, and grill for 10 to 12 minutes, until the salmon flakes with light pressure from your finger.

4. Top the salmon with the cucumbers, and garnish with a sprinkling of sesame seeds.

Makes 2 servings

Per serving: 295 cal, 36 g pro, 8 g carb, 12 g fat, 2 g sat fat, 94 mg chol, 2 g fiber, 154 mg sodium

Exchanges: ½ fat, 4½ meat, 1 vegetable

Salmon with Eggplant Mash and Pomegranate Vinaigrette

See photo insert.

2	cups yogurt		1	small onion, diced
3	tablespoons honey			Juice of 1 lemon
2	tablespoons lemon juice		2	tablespoons chopped shallots
2	tablespoons tandoori spice		2	tablespoons sliced green onions
2	tablespoons chopped fresh ginger		2	tablespoons pomegranate juice
1	pound salmon, cut into four 4-ounce pieces, bones removed		1	tablespoon brown sugar
				Seeds from ½ pomegranate
3	eggplants		1	tablespoon orange juice
2	tablespoons vegetable stock		2	tablespoons extra virgin olive oil

1. In a small bowl, whisk together the yogurt, honey, lemon juice, tandoori spice, and ginger. Pour over the salmon in a shallow baking dish and refrigerate for 4 hours.

2. Char the eggplants in a skillet for 30 minutes until soft. (The outsides should be burned.) Set aside to cool.

3. Remove the salmon and dry with a paper towel.

4. Preheat the grill. Spritz the preheated grill with cooking spray.

5. Grill the salmon until medium, 4 minutes per side.

6. Meanwhile, scoop out the eggplant pulp, chop, and sauté in a pan in the stock with onion and lemon juice until a chunky mash forms.

7. In a small bowl, whisk together the shallots, green onions, pomegranate juice, brown sugar, pomegranate seeds, orange juice, and oil. Place the salmon on the mash, then top with the vinaigrette.

Makes 4 servings

Per serving: 446 cal, 28 g pro, 42 g carb, 20 g fat, 4 g sat fat, 69 mg chol, 12 g fiber, 214 mg sodium

Exchanges: ½ fruit, ½ other carbohydrate, 2 fat, 3 meat, 4 vegetable

Mahi Mahi Wraps

4	mahi mahi fillets (6 ounces each)
1	teaspoon extra virgin olive oil
	Lemon-pepper seasoning
1	cup plain yogurt
	Juice of 2 limes
	Freshly ground black pepper
8	large leaves Boston lettuce
2	tomatoes, chopped
1	cucumber, seeded and grated
1	avocado, peeled and chopped
1	cup bean sprouts
1	cup shredded carrots

1. Heat a very clean, oiled grill or grill pan to medium.

2. Brush the fish with the oil and sprinkle it with seasoning to taste. Grill the fish, undisturbed, for 5 minutes. Carefully flip with a spatula and cook for another 5 minutes, until the fish flakes easily.

3. In a small bowl, combine the yogurt and lime juice and season to taste with black pepper. Fill each lettuce leaf with about 2 tablespoons each of the tomatoes, cucumber, avocado, sprouts, and carrots. Top each with several chunks of mahi mahi. Drizzle each with an equal amount of the yogurt sauce. Fold each lettuce leaf into a wrap.

Makes 4 servings

Per serving: 295 cal, 37 g pro, 18 g carb, 9 g fat, 2 g sat fat, 125 mg chol, 6 g fiber, 213 mg sodium

Exchanges: ½ milk, ½ fruit, 1½ fat, 1½ vegetable, 4½ very lean meat

Costa Rican–Style Snapper with Pineapple, Black Beans, and Rice

¾   cup uncooked long-grain brown rice

4   tablespoons orange juice

2   tablespoons lime juice

2   tablespoons olive oil

4   tablespoons finely chopped cilantro, divided

2   cloves garlic, minced

1   pinch sugar

   Salt

   Freshly ground black pepper

4   snapper fillets (5 ounces each), rinsed and patted dry

1   cup medium salsa

1   can (15 ounces) no-salt-added black beans, drained and rinsed

2   cups chopped pineapple

1. Preheat the oven to 400°F.

2. Cook the rice according to the package directions. Set aside.

3. In a large, shallow bowl, combine the orange and lime juices, oil, 2 tablespoons of the cilantro, garlic, and sugar, plus salt and pepper to taste. Add the snapper and marinate for 15 to 20 minutes.

4. In a 3-quart baking dish, combine the rice, salsa, beans, pineapple, and 1 tablespoon of the remaining cilantro. Place the snapper over the mixture, overlapping the fillets if necessary. Spoon the remaining marinade over the snapper.

5. Bake uncovered until the fish is cooked through and opaque, about 25 to 30 minutes. Sprinkle the remaining cilantro on top.

Makes 4 servings

Per serving: 466 cal, 37 g pro, 54 g carbs, 10 g fat, 2 g sat fat, 53 mg chol, 5 g fiber, 594 mg sodium

Exchanges: 2½ starch, ½ fruit, 1½ fat, 1 vegetable, 4 very lean meat

Grilled Spicy Fish Tacos

1	mango, peeled, pitted, and cubed
1	avocado, peeled, pitted, and cubed
½	medium red onion, diced
1	handful cilantro, chopped
2	limes
	Salt
	Freshly ground black pepper
	Canola oil
12	ounces mahi mahi
½	tablespoon blackening spice
4	corn tortillas
1	cup finely shredded red cabbage

1. Clean and oil a grill or grill pan thoroughly. Preheat to medium-high.

2. In a medium bowl, combine the mango, avocado, red onion, cilantro, and the juice of one lime. Season to taste with salt and pepper.

3. Drizzle a light coating of oil over the fish, and rub on the blackening spice. Grill the fish undisturbed for 4 minutes. Carefully flip with a spatula and cook for another 4 minutes. Remove. Before turning off the grill, warm the tortillas directly on the surface for 1 to 2 minutes.

4. Divide the fish evenly among the warm tortillas, add a bit of cabbage, and spoon the salsa on top. Serve each taco with a wedge of lime.

Makes 2 servings

Per serving: 571 cal, 38 g pro, 62 g carb, 23 g fat, 3 g sat fat, 124 mg chol, 15 g fiber, 891 mg sodium

Exchanges: 1½ starch, 2 fruit, 4 fat, 1 vegetable, 4½ very lean meat

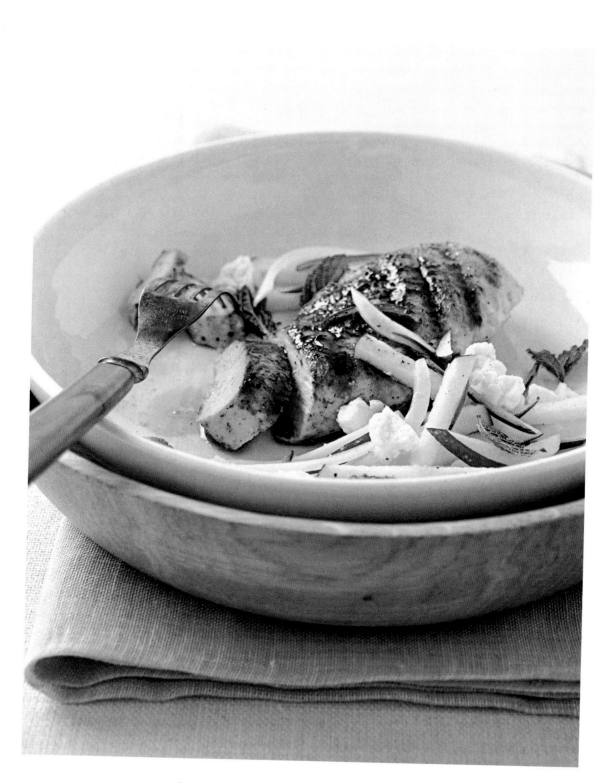

Grilled Chicken with Goat Cheese and Apples
Recipe on page 313

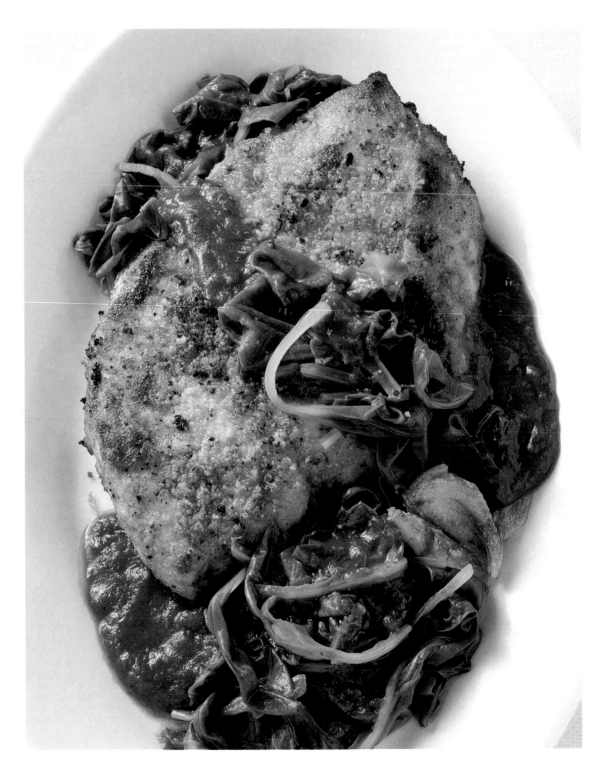

Chicken Spinach Parm
Recipe on page 314

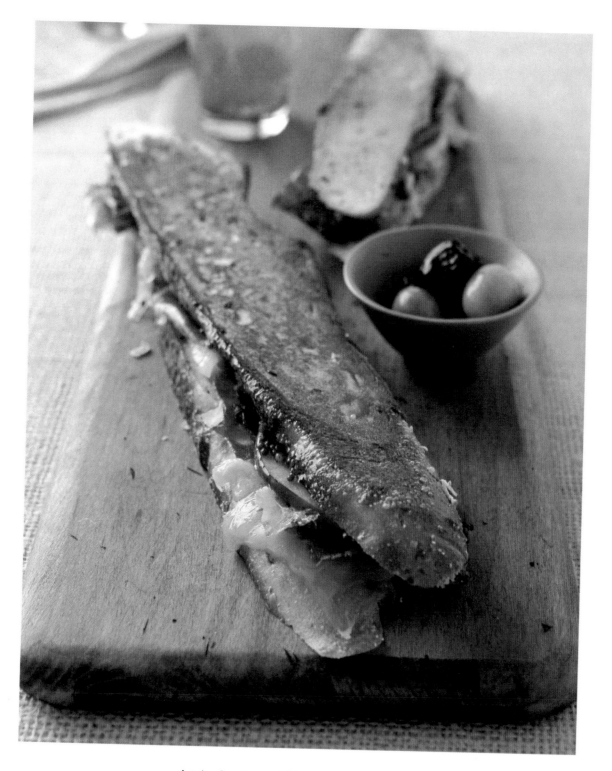

Apple, Gouda, and Crispy Prosciutto Panini
Recipe on page 322

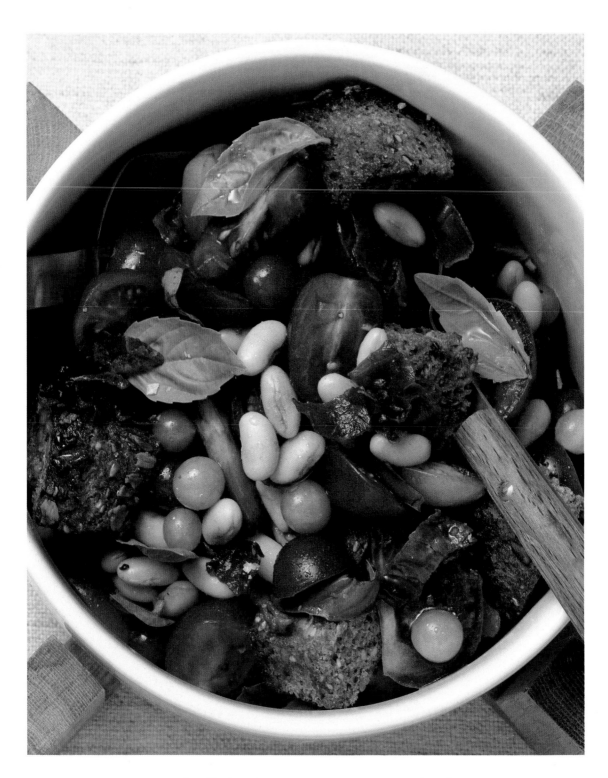

Panzanella with Tomatoes, White Beans, Basil, and Prosciutto
Recipe on page 323

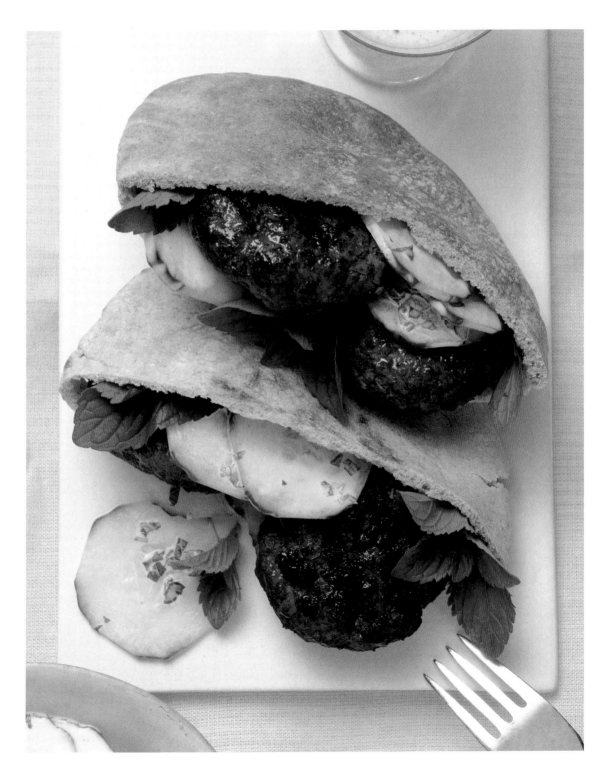

Mini Pita Burgers with Cucumber Mint Salad
Recipe on page 327

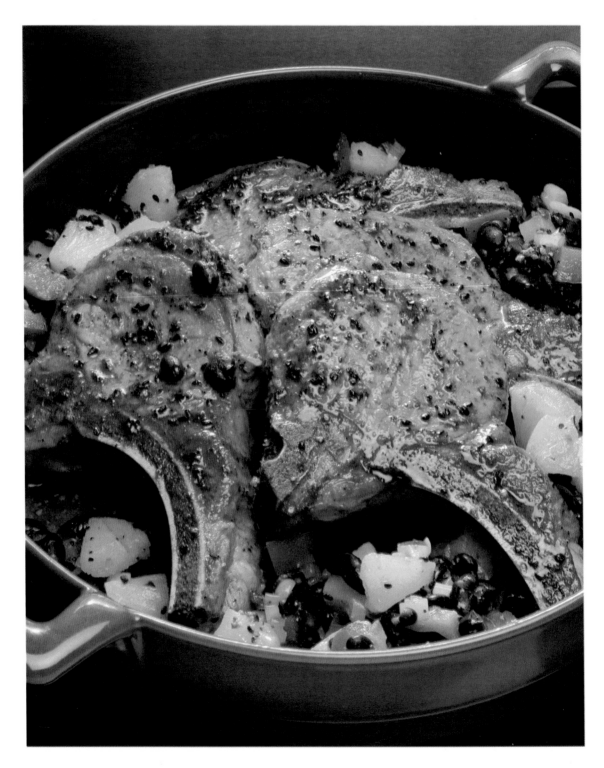

Jerk Pork with Pineapple and Black Beans
Recipe on page 329

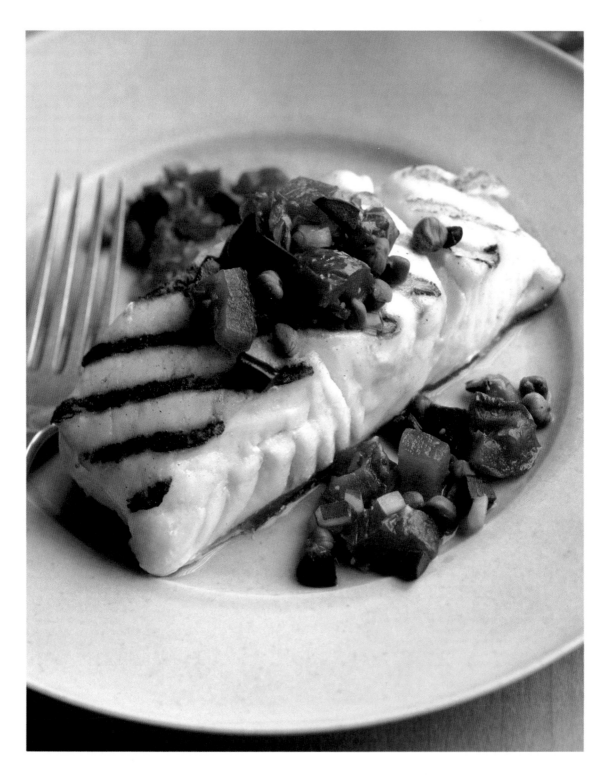

Grilled Halibut with Roasted-Tomato Tapenade
Recipe on page 335

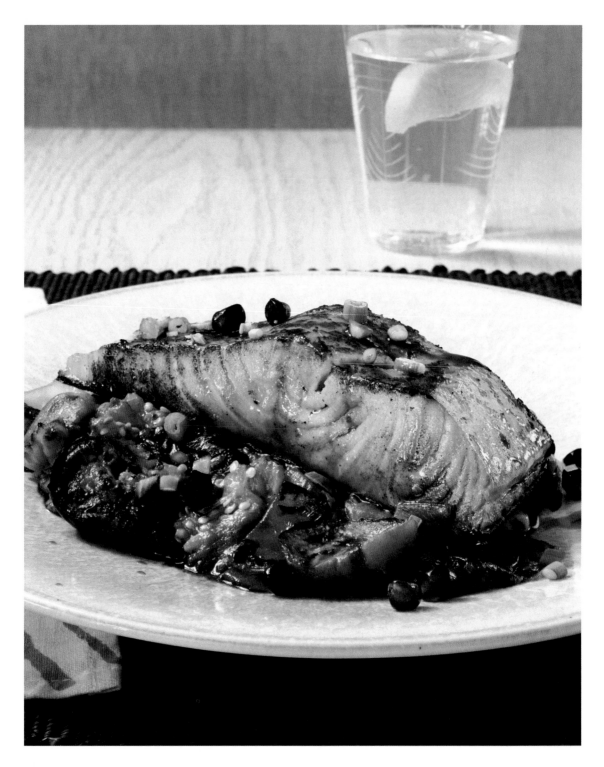

Salmon with Eggplant Mash and Pomegranate Vinaigrette
Recipe on page 339

Heart-Healthy Burger

10	ounces ahi tuna, divided into two portions
	Olive oil
	Salt
	Freshly ground black pepper
2	ciabatta or focaccia rolls, toasted
2	tablespoons prepared pesto
2	tablespoons mayonnaise
1	tomato, sliced
¼	red onion, thinly sliced
2	cups mixed greens

1. Preheat the grill.

2. Coat the tuna with the oil and season with salt and pepper to taste. Grill on high heat for 2 minutes per side, until the outside is lightly charred but the interior is still pink and cool.

3. Toast the buns and top with the pesto and mayonnaise. Divide the tomato, onion, and greens between the two buns. Place one piece of tuna on each bun.

Makes 2 servings

Per serving: 476 cal, 42 g pro, 41 g carb, 16 g fat, 3 g sat fat, 73 mg chol, 4 g fiber, 692 mg sodium

Exchanges: 2 starch, 2½ fat, ½ meat, 1½ vegetable, 4½ very lean meat

Spicy Garlic Shrimp

1	tablespoon olive oil
1	tablespoon red-pepper flakes
4	cloves garlic, thinly sliced
1	pound shrimp, peeled and deveined
	Salt
	Ground black pepper
1	tablespoon chopped parsley

1. In a small sauté pan, heat the oil until it starts to simmer (just below smoking temperature). Add the pepper flakes and then the garlic.

2. Meanwhile, season the shrimp with salt and black pepper, then place the shrimp in the pan with the garlic, swirling the pan gently. Sauté over medium-high heat for 1 minute, then stir in the parsley. Sauté for another minute.

Makes 4 servings

Per serving: 155 cal, 23 g pro, 2 g carb, 5 g fat, 1 g sat fat, 172 mg chol, 0.14 g fiber, 242 mg sodium

Exchanges: 1 fat, 3½ very lean meat

Roasted Shrimp 'n Vegetable Pasta

1	pound large raw shrimp, peeled and deveined
1	cup white wine
$\frac{1}{2}$	teaspoon red-pepper flakes
$\frac{1}{4}$	teaspoon freshly ground black pepper + more to taste
4	cloves garlic, minced
2	medium yellow squash, cubed
12–15	asparagus stalks, stemmed and cut into 2" pieces
12	grape or cherry tomatoes
2	teaspoons olive oil
$\frac{1}{2}$	box penne pasta, cooked
1	tablespoon flax oil
4–5	fresh basil leaves, chopped
4	teaspoons grated Parmesan cheese

1. In a large ziplock bag, add the shrimp, wine, red pepper, black pepper, and garlic. Marinate in the refrigerator for 1 hour.

2. Preheat the broiler.

3. In a baking pan, mix the squash, asparagus, and tomatoes, and toss with a bit of olive oil and black pepper. Place 6 inches from the heat in the oven. Broil for 5 minutes, and remove. Add the shrimp to the pan, and broil for $2\frac{1}{2}$ minutes. Spoon the shrimp and vegetables over the hot pasta. Add the flax oil, basil, and Parmesan, then toss.

Makes 4 servings

Per serving: 377 cal, 30 g pro, 32 g carb, 9 g fat, 1 g sat fat, 174 mg chol, 4 g fiber, 200 mg sodium

Exchanges: 1½ starch, 1½ fat, 1½ vegetable, 3½ very lean meat

Cajun Shrimp Sandwich and Green Gazpacho

3	cucumbers, peeled and chopped		1	teaspoon paprika
½	cup loosely packed basil leaves		1–2	pinches salt
½	cup chopped green bell pepper		1	tablespoon olive oil
1	clove garlic		1	large onion, sliced
1	cup low-sodium chicken broth		1	large red bell pepper, seeded and sliced lengthwise
1	cup low-fat Greek-style yogurt (We used Fage Total 2 percent.)		1–2	tablespoons water
1	pound jumbo shrimp, peeled and deveined		1	large whole wheat baguette, sliced in half lengthwise and cut into four 5" pieces
1	tablespoon salt-free Cajun spice			
1	teaspoon dried garlic			

1. Preheat the oven to 400°F.

2. In a blender, puree the cucumber, basil, bell pepper, garlic, and broth until smooth. Pour into a bowl. Whisk in the yogurt, cover, and place in the freezer.

3. In a medium bowl, toss the shrimp with the Cajun spice, garlic, paprika, and salt and set aside.

4. In a large nonstick saucepan, heat the oil on medium-high. Add the onion and pepper and sauté, shaking the pan, until softened, for 4 to 5 minutes. Add the water and continue cooking for 3 to 4 minutes.

5. Turn the heat up to high, add the shrimp, and sauté until pink, about 3 minutes.

6. Hollow out the baguette pieces, leaving only crust. Place on a baking sheet and toast in the oven until the crust is crispy, 2 to 3 minutes.

7. To assemble, place ¼ of the shrimp-onion mixture on each baguette bottom and cover with baguette top. Serve with the cold gazpacho.

Makes 4 servings

Per serving: 335 cal, 31 g pro, 33 g carb, 8 g fat, 2 g sat fat, 160 mg chol, 5 g fiber, 493 mg sodium

Exchanges: 1 starch, 1 fat, 2 vegetable, 3 very lean meat

Seared Scallops over Buckwheat Noodles with Honey Yuzu Vinaigrette

16	diver scallops	$\frac{1}{3}$	cup yuzu or rice vinegar
	Salt	3	tablespoons low-sodium soy sauce
	Freshly ground black pepper	2	tablespoons honey
8	ounces buckwheat noodles	1	teaspoon lemon juice
$\frac{3}{4}$	cup water	1	teaspoon olive oil
3	tablespoons (or tea bags) buckwheat tea	$\frac{1}{2}$	pound sugar snap peas, sliced on bias
5	tablespoons olive oil	2	cups cherry tomatoes, halved

1. Season the scallops with salt and pepper and set aside.

2. Tie the noodles together at one end with a rubber band and cook according to the package directions. When finished, cut the hard ends of the noodles off.

3. Meanwhile, bring the water to a boil. Remove from the heat, add the tea, and let steep for 5 minutes. Strain the tea and whisk in the oil, vinegar, soy sauce, honey, lemon juice, and pepper to taste.

4. Place the noodles in a medium bowl. Coat the noodles with the vinaigrette, saving some to coat the peas and tomatoes later, and let stand.

5. In a pan, heat the oil and sear the scallops for $1\frac{1}{2}$ minutes on each side. (Spread them out so they cook evenly.) Remove the scallops from the pan and place on a paper towel.

6. Blanch the peas by dunking them into boiling water briefly, then place them in a bowl of cold water.

7. To serve, pinch a bunch of noodles and arrange in a swirl on each dish, topping with four scallops per serving. Place the peas and tomatoes on the side or sprinkle them over the scallops and noodles. Drizzle with the reserved dressing.

Makes 4 servings

Per serving: 492 cal, 19 g pro, 62 g carb, 20 g fat, 3 g sat fat, 20 mg chol, 5 g fiber, 605 mg sodium

Exchanges: 2½ starch, ½ other carbohydrate, 3½ fat, 1½ vegetable, 1½ very lean meat

Garlic and Tomato Mussels

1	teaspoon extra virgin olive oil
1	small yellow onion, chopped
2	cloves garlic, minced
2	dozen mussels
$\frac{1}{2}$	cup water
1	cup dry white wine
1	large tomato, chopped
2	tablespoons chopped fresh parsley

1. In a large pot, heat the oil over medium heat. Add the onion and garlic, and sauté until lightly browned. Then add the mussels, water, and wine. Reduce the heat to low and cover with a lid. (After 3 to 4 minutes, the mussels will begin to open.) Remove the lid, add the tomato and parsley, and cover again for 1 minute.

2. Transfer the mussels to two large bowls and spoon on some of the sauce from the pot.

Makes 2 servings

Per serving: 258 cal, 16 g pro, 15 g carb, 5 g fat, 1 g sat fat, 134 mg chol, 2 g fiber, 354 mg sodium

Exchanges: ½ fat, 2 meat, 1½ vegetable

photograph credits

Photo Insert # 1 (starts with Whole Wheat French Toast with Pumpkin Butter)

    pages 1 and 6: © Romulo Yanes

    page 2: © Ellie Miller

    page 3: © Kristen Strecker

    pages 4 and 5: © Sang An

    page 7: © Mitch Mandel/Rodale Images

    page 8: © Scott Peterson

Photo Insert #2 (starts with Grilled Chicken with Goat Cheese and Apples)

    pages 1 and 3: © Kristen Strecker

    page 2: © Tim Turner

    pages 4 and 5: © Jonathan Kantor

    page 6: © Hans Gissinger

    page 7: © Catherine Sears

    page 8: © Jeff Harris

Exercise Photos

    pages 141–146, 156–166: © David Martinez

    pages 150–154, 169–176: © John Dolan

INDEX

Underscored page references indicate boxed text and tables. **Boldface** references indicate photographs. An asterisk (*) indicates recipe photos are shown in the color inserts.